Early Childhood Development

Early Childhood Development

From understanding to initiatives ...

EDITOR
Bilal Iqbal Avan

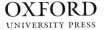
OXFORD
UNIVERSITY PRESS

OXFORD
UNIVERSITY PRESS

Great Clarendon Street, Oxford ox2 6dp

Oxford University Press is a department of the University of Oxford.
It furthers the University's objective of excellence in research, scholarship,
and education by publishing worldwide in

Oxford New York

Auckland Cape Town Dar es Salaam Hong Kong Karachi
Kuala Lumpur Madrid Melbourne Mexico City Nairobi
New Delhi Shanghai Taipei Toronto

with offices in

Argentina Austria Brazil Chile Czech Republic France Greece
Guatemala Hungary Italy Japan Poland Portugal Singapore
South Korea Switzerland Turkey Ukraine Vietnam

Oxford is a registered trade mark of Oxford University Press
in the UK and in certain other countries

ISBN 978-0-19-547597-5

Typeset in Optima
Printed in Pakistan by
Mas Printers, Karachi.
Published by
Ameena Saiyid, Oxford University Press
No. 38, Sector 15, Korangi Industrial Area, PO Box 8214
Karachi-74900, Pakistan.

CONTENTS

FOREWORD

Although the child survival revolution of the 1980s achieved a dramatic decrease in the number of children who die before reaching their fifth birthday, much remains to be done. There are still more than 10 million childhood deaths a year; most countries are not on track to reach the Millennium Development Goal for child health: to reduce by 2015 the level of child mortality by two thirds of its level in 1990. The problem is not lack of knowledge; the authors of the seminal Lancet child survival series published in 2003 estimated that two-thirds of childhood deaths could be prevented by ensuring universal coverage with a handful of simple measures. They called for a second child survival revolution, and threw down a challenge to governments, international and bi-lateral agencies and health care professionals to act promptly. We have an ethical imperative; we must not continue to fail to meet our obligations to the children of the world in this way.

Tackling child survival is, however, not enough. Poor children of the world bear a double burden. Childhood deaths are only the tip of the iceberg; millions of children that survive do so in sub-optimal circumstances. Many suffer from developmental disabilities such as: specific learning disabilities, visual or hearing disabilities, motor disabilities, language disorders or behavioural disorders. In many countries, the majority of these children currently go unrecognised and therefore fail to receive any of the health, social or educational interventions that might mitigate the impact of the developmental disability. Even more children survive with no obvious specific disability, but suffer from developmental delay or sub-optimal growth, with poor children being disproportionately affected. Although no data currently exist on the exact number, it is known that about 40% of children in developing countries are growth retarded by their fifth birthday. Millions of children currently fail to reach their full developmental potential; this has a profound impact on their educational achievement and employment opportunities later in life.

Improving child survival is therefore only one aspect of fulfilling our obligations to the children of the world; ensuring the quality of their survival is equally important, but unfortunately often neglected. Currently, less than a third of children benefit from any form of early childhood education, compared to about 80% in many countries in Europe; in much of sub-Saharan Africa, only 1% of eligible children are enrolled in preschool programmes. An even smaller proportion currently benefit from the broader developmental strategies shown to be effective in the first years of life.

The publication of this book is most timely and welcome; it fills an important gap and should appeal to a wide audience. Early child development is a relatively new initiative in much of the developing world, there is a general lack of trained personnel and few programmes have comprehensively tackled this gap. Many caregivers do not know what is needed to enable children to thrive when they are living in poor and deprived environments, subject to frequent episodes of illness and inadequate diet.

The book starts with a detailed theoretical account of child development and the role that the social environment plays in this. It then outlines the different tools and instruments to assess a child's development, and provides guidance for health personnel on how to give advice to caregivers to encourage actions to promote child growth and development. It also discusses the relevance and content of community-based initiatives to promote holistic child development. Last but not least, the book includes a detailed structure for the outline of a training course, with learning objectives for a number of teaching sessions drawing on material presented in the book, and advice on teaching methods to be used. This is designed in a way to enable the sessions to be customised to make them culturally and linguistically appropriate.

I would like to congratulate Dr Bilal Iqbal Avan and all the contributors not only for the comprehensive content and thoughtful approach, but also for the small touches that inspire us as we read the book, in particular the wide-ranging and optimistic quotes and the delightful children's paintings that introduce each chapter. I believe this book will prove of great benefit not only in the training of specialised child development personnel and in improving the knowledge and skills of primary care personnel, but also in helping parents to understand what children need. It gives hope that it is possible to create environments in which all children can thrive whatever their circumstances.

Betty Kirkwood
Professor of Epidemiology and International Health
London School of Hygiene and Tropical Medicine,
London

PREFACE

Childhood is an endearing phase of life for the child as well as for the family. In addition, it has the potential to create hope of happiness and prosperity for the community and nations at large. The critical significance of the early phase of life is not only highlighted in the conventional wisdoms but also proven by modern scientific facts generated by behavioural, economic, and medical and social sciences. Soundly nurtured children yield physically developed persons, psycho-socially stable personalities, cognitively and economically productive citizens, and above all, a responsible and conscientious society.

"It takes a village to raise a child", this African logic has universal appeal in terms of defining the role of caregivers and community, and integration of all systems and services to accomplish a common perspective of achieving better developed children. Unfortunately, productive and meaningful experience of Early Childhood Development (ECD) has been turned into a tragedy for millions of children around the globe especially from the developing countries. In the context of under-nutrition and neglect, they are never able to achieve their full potentials and productivities during their adulthood; creating a vicious cycle of poverty and underprivileged societies. This devastating effect is multifaceted in origin involving inter-related factors, and poverty or lack of resources cannot be the only factor to be blamed.

Today, more and more nations around the world are recognizing that the major challenge is lack of adequately skilled and knowledgeable caregivers as well as optimal functioning and integration of services available at community level. Policy makers and financing organizations increasingly value ECD, but require empirical evidence and change of perspective to proceed further. The dilemma is the architecture of a conducive environment for child development, which is global in its nature, rather than linear or hierarchical in terms of its diverse components. Each factor has its own unique place and significance, thus advocating a case of comprehensive environment for holistic development. A critical challenge for ECD is to trounce those impediments that prevent the application of the broad array of available preventive strategies. These needs and concerns served as the impetus for the book. The title "Early Childhood Development — from understanding to initiatives" points to not only the extensive range of issues but also the arrangements nations make to deal with them. The unique feature of this book is that explanations from diverse disciplines have been synthesized in order to explain a solitary consistent framework. The purpose is to create a universal language for thinking, communication and action regarding ECD.

Fundamentally, the book is developed by focusing two types of relevant audience. Specifically, the ideas in this book cut across students, caregivers including ECD practitioners, organizations, and functional specialties (Education, Health, Social Sciences). But generally it also addresses the layman who is concerned about a better future of his / her children. The book is organized in a manner to allow the reader a direct, concise and jargon free approach to the subject. The purpose is that irrespective of one's status or responsibilities in terms of ECD, one must be able to understand the relation between community and the child development cycle; appreciate determinants, practice assessment techniques, interpret and communicate the growth and development status, advocate the basic ECD arguments, pursue collective thinking, ability to plan and solve problems, manage their children and expertise to work with the organizations and communities to accomplish ECD endeavours in a culturally appropriate way.

We are optimistic that this book will be an informative, gratifying and inspirational reading experience for its readers. Even if a few of our readers get the motivation and expertise, and opt for professions and vocations that save the children from harm and support ECD in its true spirit, our cause would be achieved. We will believe that we have been successful.

Bilal Iqbal Avan

ACKNOWLEDGEMENTS

An achievement at this level is not possible without a sincere and supportive social system. I feel fortunate enough being blessed with encouraging and compassionate individuals who, professionally and personally, enriched me in my cause for ECD.

I would first of all like to thank Camer W Villani for stimulating me to work on human development through child development. I consider myself honoured to have the opportunity to learn from his value system, especially demonstration of logic, rigour and dedication to the profession. Above all I would like to express gratitude to him for being my mentor, and being there for me whenever I needed guidance or clarity of vision. In the same spirit, Franklin C White is another visionary in my career who believed in me, inspired me and supported my career in Public Health and ECD. I have tremendous gratitude for both of them. I also happen to be endowed with sincere and warm-hearted friends. Haroon Afridi, Qazi Jibran and Arshad Altaf supported my endeavour and stance through all possible means. I have the deepest of respect for this relationship and a profound appreciation of their camaraderie. Naushaba Mobeen is another special person of exceptional wit and intellect. I have been privileged to have discussions with her on various issues and challenges, and benefited from her optimistic perspective. I also value Adnan Hameed for his unconditional support at personal as well as professional level. The role of Razia Asifali (my assistant) needs special mention for her logistical support, and also for keeping me organised and disciplined.

I acknowledge the cooperation of the International Maternal and Child Health Research Training (IMCHRT) program from the Fogarty International Centre, USA and University Research Council of Aga Khan University (URC, AKU), Pakistan. In this regard, I would like to mention here the keen interest shown in this publication by Sibylle Kristensen (IMCHRT, University of Alabama at Birmingham, USA), Nasiruddin Muhammad Ali (CHS, AKU) and Anwar Siddique (URC, AKU). Support of these persons and organizations is admiringly recognized.

In the end, I would like to ask forgiveness for not being able to mention the names of all the individuals, who directly or indirectly were part of this challenging/momentous task.

Bilal Iqbal Avan

INTRODUCTION

Early Childhood Development...

Definition

The domains of ECD consist of intellectual, physical and social development of young children. During the process of development, disturbance in one domain affects the other domains. Therefore, child development is a continuous process of maintaining equilibrium between various domains to achieve an optimal level of physical and economical efficiency of a human being, with psycho-socially acceptable features.

Situation

Traditionally, families and communities have formed beliefs and practices regarding provision, security, shelter, clothing, hygiene and feeding needs of younger children. Irrespective of factual status, emphasis is laid on these practices; consequently, the concept of childcare and expectations for development were narrowly focused on responding only to basic needs for survival and physical growth.

There has been no conscious effort towards recognising meaningful interaction and stimulation as a child's basic need, while the case of linking investment during early childhood to achieve greater assets of human development in the future is also missing. The obvious dilemma at family, community and even country level is to consider why and what to invest, and what to expect in terms of optimal growth and development during early childhood.

This vision of child development is further augmented by the prevalent service provision infrastructure and community development projects, which are again focused on narrowed vision, emphasizing mainly physical growth and survival rather than the whole concept of child development and care. The primary reason for this publication is ease in demonstration of change in a child's physical growth, morbidity and mortality, as evidenced by changing indicators. These changes are also reflected in a child's holistic development, including social and intellectual aspects, which also require relatively more insight, rigor, resources and especially – commitment.

In addition, standards and expectations of intellectual and social development are based on the local cultural perspective as opposed to standards of physical development that are universally accepted and used for comparison.

Concept

Modern literature in the discipline of child development is concentrated in two domains in an integrated manner; it includes processes of child development and environment which influences the pace and modification of such processes. Any effort to lift the status of children requires proper philosophical underpinnings of both.

It is important to expand the prevailing narrow concept of mere child survival to quality of survival. This implies the process of enabling the child to reach the broader pedestal of human performance in society, and development of expertise and skills which contribute to social competency.

'It takes a village to raise a child'; this African proverb is valid for every culture because it highlights the significance of responsibilities and collective function of the community to nurture their children. Child and family units are always implanted in the larger socio-economic and cultural framework of the community. This framework has all the potential to influence functioning of the family unit, especially the process of child development, by availability of necessary persons, places or resources, e.g., schools, playgrounds, health care systems etc. This contextual outline is vital for continuum of the conceptual understanding of ECD to facilitate execution of initiatives at individual and communal level. The entire book is distinctively focused on the theoretical framework of "Ecology of Human Development" suggested by Urie Bronfenbrenner; child development is primarily influenced by the child's interaction with the critical elements of the environment, which extend from family to neighbourhood, community services, social institutions, and socio-cultural conditions. The perspective of critical elements of the social environment is throughout maintained in the descriptions of the processes involving child development as well as methods and actions required for optimal child development and growth.

Understanding

In ECD, a culturally contextualized approach leads to better understanding of specific dynamics and expectations. At the family level, critical elements of the social environment can be identified; the configuration is unique for each individual child, while at the community level, appreciation of its concepts of achieving more productive and responsible members is developed. It requires information at three levels i.e. status of prevailing childcare and nurturing practices, their effects on growth and development, and understanding of the basis for cultural practices.

In order to progress and achieve holistic child development and care, it is important that ECD projects shift from authoritarian and dictated approaches of following global standards of certain limited aspects of child development, which expect conformity for every child, (e.g., optimal height and weight), irrespective of cultural, ecological and even genetic differences. Currently, the need for such a paradigm shift is clearly needed by practitioners in the field of child development.

Initiatives

ECD is a broad based scientific discipline with its roots in medical, behavioural and social sciences. Consequently, an ECD practitioner requires broad based knowledge as well as skills. In addition, ECD requires purposeful and well-designed integration of relevant services to achieve holistic child development. However, for all practical purposes, the public health system due to its diversity and multi-sectoral nature, and overlapping interest seems most closely linked with ECD to develop initiatives for child development. The theoretical framework of all the relevant disciplines needs to be considered primarily under the umbrella of Public Health, so that ideas can reach the stage of practical implementation, and can become components of the service delivery system, thus keeping its feasibility, multiplicity and integrity intact.

The book...

The idea here is not to create a comprehensive text, especially in the context of knowledge, when ECD as a discipline is evolving fast. Discipline-specific details about child development can be found in the relevant advanced texts. The purpose here is to create a unifying set of ideas of balanced views, to address the core issues of younger children in developing countries, which is conceptually acceptable to all disciplines without overpowering any one of them. The scheme is to create generic guidelines for the relevant ECD practitioner, for understanding the concept of ECD, determining its stature and interventions in speeding the process of child development

The book has been compiled with the perspective of human capacity building for ECD endeavours. From household to professional ECD practitioners, any organised effort to improve the status of young children requires understanding at multiple levels, apart from compassion for the cause. The design of the book has considered the following framework to facilitate the progress of the reader from understanding to initiatives. The fundamental assumptions of each step of this hierarchical paradigm are important for the understanding of theoretical knowledge from the viewpoint of its utility; the effort has been to achieve a harmonious blend of theory and practice.

1. The conceptual framework of ECD is primarily predetermined by the human genetic potential, but the pace and extent of developmental achievements is determined by the environment. This leads to an understanding of expectation from the child in terms of age-appropriate growth and development. In addition, the extended role of caregivers for their relative control over the environment is envisaged.

2. Critical elements of the social environment, which influence ECD outcomes, include the child's interactions with family and community, and the socioeconomic and cultural context in which these interactions take place. This scenario highlights the interaction of ECD stakeholders with a variety of disciplines. It leads to multiple avenues of intervention and prevention, as well as numerous combinations of partnerships to achieve holistic child development.

3. Appropriate scientific assessment, both quantitative and qualitative, is based on determination of the status of growth and development of the child. Any evidence regarding the individual or communal status requires diligent and judicious quantitative estimation of performance to make that information eligible for the decision-making process. The systematic process of measuring is a prerequisite for comparison of the child's status with the additional resources required for remedial action. This in turn implies that the data generation and interpretation capacity of any ECD endeavour is imperative.

4. Child assessment should always be accompanied by a proposal for an appropriate course of action. For ECD practitioners, it is a component of their responsibilities by virtue of their position; provision of comprehensive advice of guided actions for the caregiver for further improvement, and remedial activities.

5. Child-centred community development approach is vital for lasting solutions for the child's as well as the community's prosperity. It is the capacity building of people to recognize their requirements and priorities, and to seek solution for their own community development through focussed achievement of holistic child development. It is important for ECD practitioners to realize that such investment by the community is necessary to improve the existing state of social and economic deprivation, and ensure that improvement on a permanent basis. This philosophy encompasses participation, empowerment, equity and social justice for every vulnerable subgroup of the community.

6. Diversity in involved child caregivers is imperative. Despite equal significance of each of them, their capacity to contribute varies; programming mechanism is evolved through public health to train the stakeholders and integrate their efforts to bring efficient child development.

The contents...

The book primarily has four (4) thematic parts, which form the basis of chapters related to respective themes. The continuum has been maintained from development of basic understanding of the discipline to transformation of theory into practice, in order to facilitate a learner in confidently taking ECD related initiatives.

Part A - Core Concepts: The objective of this part is to introduce theoretical concepts of childhood developmental milestones and underlying philosophy of interactions of the child with the social environment. **Chapter 1** provides a comprehensive review of the premise of early childhood development, by focusing on appreciation of basic definitions and concepts of growth and developmental domains during this phase. It concludes with a discussion on various factors affecting child development. **Chapter 2** examines the context in which child development takes place by addressing the potential role of sensory stimulation in growth and development, and its relationship with the social environment. In addition, it explores various considerations for caregivers to evaluate the qualitative aspects of the social environment for its capacity to stimulate a child.

Part B – Assessments and Advice: The purpose of this section is to outline the technical skills and expertise necessary to assess the processes and status of child development. The explanation of methodologies is kept simple but scientific enough for use in any professional and/or non-professional avenues, including community-based settings. Acquisition of assessment skills without any guidance for further action is not going to bring any meaningful change in the status of children. Therefore, feasible suggestions for possible actions are provided along with assessment methodologies, to promote the growth and developmental status of the child. **Chapter 3** presents the general guidelines and prerequisites for child assessment. The focus is on rapport building from the perspective of an assessor. Conceptual understanding of a child's nature in terms of personality and temperament has been described as the potential consideration for any type of assessment. **Chapter 4** introduces the several echelons of nutrition, one of the primary concerns for child development in any resource-scarce setting. Discussion is on the understanding of nutrients, balanced diet and alternate sources of nutrition. Differential nutritional needs of pregnancy and the early childhood period are also highlighted. The chapter then presents a detailed account of anthropometric measurement, and its significance for decision making at individual and programmatic levels. **Chapter 5** begins by explaining the concepts of intelligence with emphasis on contribution of hereditary and environmental factors. Reflection on the relationship between intelligence and learning including some of the challenges encountered during the learning process of a child (such as learning styles and disability) are presented. **Chapter 6** then begins with a brief overview of scientific observation and the importance of its contextualization to obtain an inclusive analysis. Observational skills have marked implication for the identification of child-rearing practices, in particular care and nurturance, which require modification and promotion; this is exemplified further with examples of parent and child behaviour, such as parenting styles, play, reinforcement and punishment. **Chapter 7** is dedicated to interviewing skills with special consideration on development of questionnaire and guidelines for conducting the interview process in a community setting. Additional information is also provided on the methodology to identify the eligible interviewees. **Chapter 8** covers the comparison of focus group discussions with other forms of scientific inquiry and its process. The focus group discussions are then linked with detailed accounts of positive deviance inquiry. This is an inquiry into the reasons for positive deviation from regular child rearing practices, which result in more than expected growth and developmental status of the child. In addition, the process facilitates the implementation of intervention of identified practices through community mobilization and participation. **Chapter 9** examines the basic components and domains of communication. Consideration is also given to the communication skills of ECD practitioners for formal interactions. Apart from interviews, attention is drawn to the importance of counselling of caregivers for provision of information and guidance, with persuasion to adopt a more conducive attitude and practices for child development.

Part C - ECD Community Based Programming:
The objective of this section is to familiarize ECD practitioners with community-based ECD programming, with application of the planning cycle to the stage of conceptualization, implementation and management of ECD community-based projects. We believe that the process of providing care and a supportive environment for children is learnt through experience and therefore, we do not have a model to describe it, nor do we recommend its adoption by others. The assumption is that individual practitioners would act as resource persons for their specific community set-up. Within the limits of its context and resources, they will be able to successfully develop and implement ECD model activities. **Chapter 10** deals with the understanding of community dynamics from the perspective of ECD. Principles for community orientation as well as selection of the appropriate community for ECD-related initiatives are outlined. **Chapter 11** introduces the concept of community-based ECD programming; the planning cycle with all its components has been discussed in detail, from situation analysis, setting priorities and objectives to planning activities for achieving holistic child development through integrated efforts of stakeholders at community level. The remaining part of this chapter reviews the ingredients of documentation for ECD programme planning. **Chapter 12** emphasizes the actual implementation of programming concepts into practice. ECD programme management is extremely dependent on the interest of the community and their representatives. Field coordination is important for transformation of their interest into motivation towards child centred community development. Technical details of community-based programming are elaborated from team formation, capacity building, and baseline assessments, followed by monitoring and evaluation of the implemented strategies. The chapter concludes with a discussion on the documentation of programmatic activities, as this plays a significant role in reporting and dissemination of the successful endeavours.

Part D – Teaching and Training:
Capacity building of ECD practitioners is a major concern for the implementation of ECD initiatives, especially in developing country scenarios. The experiential learning approach is adopted, as it requires integration of existing skills with the newly acquired knowledge, and reflection by the learner, to assimilate and utilize that information for problem solving in his/her current context. The professional background of learners could be quite diverse, due to the multidisciplinary nature of child development itself. However, the only criteria suggested are affection, care, concern for conditions that support growth and development of children, and a sense of community responsibility. Special efforts have been made to develop training contents relevant for the caregivers, especially practitioners, as well as clear enough for trainers, so that they can be used as resource material for course planning. Teaching and training have been innovatively linked with concepts and discussion, in each of the preceding twelve chapters; objectives for the lecture session are followed by detailed accounts of an assortment of activities, to develop the attitude and skills required for an effective ECD practice.

The sessions are arranged in a specific sequence for a complete text for ECD programming. However, it is flexible enough for components to be selected according to the specific teaching and training purposes. It is recommended that the examples and instructions should be contextualized according to the respective needs of the learner. Due to the diversity of the audience who will use the text, from caregivers to practitioners to academics and students, special attention has been given to provision of sufficient information, with clear and straightforward learning objectives and plan. In theoretical content, we intentionally tried to give simple definitions and descriptions, but kept intact the abstract conceptual soul and idea of child development. In addition, the attempt has been to achieve coherence between initiatives of child development and the scope of the culture and communities for whom this book is intended.

The team...

ECD as a discipline has no rigid boundaries; care and nurturance for children involve an ever-increasing number of expertise and skills that go much beyond those expected from a conventional caregiver. Due to the multiplicity of disciplines involved, drawing together a team from varied faculties to do the collaborative task was a challenge. I was able to assemble the team by identifying the talent of some of my colleagues and students who have evolved into experts in their respective fields. They are physicians, psychologists, community health nurses, sociologists, public health practitioners, epidemiologists, and representatives of NGOs. Each member was vital in the completion of this prodigious task, and was a source of strength and support for me in the preparation of this text. Despite their important existing commitments, each of them showed dedication and lent support to the cause of ECD. I owe them sincere thanks for their passion and patience.

For organizational purposes, the team members were divided into sub-groups according to the respective themes of the book; each sub-group facilitated me in the assemblage of specific parts, based on their experience in academics, research and service.

Part A - Core Concepts: The first part of the book is primarily based on the discipline of child psychology. Being a psychologist, Bushra Khan added depth to this component, and was ably supported by Anjum Sharif.

Part B – Assessments and Advice: This part of the book best represents the disciplinary multiplicity involved in the provision of care for the child. Detailed documentation on nutrition, growth and anthropometry are the result of the efforts of Saima Akhund (Physician). The hard work of Abdul Wajid (representative of NGO, Epidemiologist) for Questionnaire Based Interviews and Tazeen Saeed Ali (Community Health Nurse, Epidemiologist) for Communication Skills is remarkable. Chapters on General Guidelines for Child Assessment, Observational Methodology, Intellectual Assessment and Focus Group Discussions provide strong evidence of the exhaustive work of Bushra Khan, along with Sanober (Psychologist), and Zeenat (Community Health Nurse).

Part C - ECD Community Based Programming: This part demonstrates the merging of the action-oriented features of Public Health and social sciences with ECD. The Community Dynamics portion is highlighted by Irum Fatima (Sociologist). Hasan Bin Hamza and Ahsan Raza (Public Health Epidemiologists) brought the ECD Programming aspect together. This duo has evolved from my students to thorough professionals and friends. I enjoyed working with them very much.

Contributors: Include those who at any occasion provided the team with valuable suggestions and comments during the write-up process. Keeping in view their expertise and consideration, I am extremely appreciative of the support. I would specially like to mention Hilda Saeed for her professional text editing: she was persistent and meticulous in subjecting the manuscript to extensive review, with particular attention to ensure that the content and language remained neutral in terms of ethnicity and gender.

Creative Arts Team: This book has been fortunate in availing the creative abilities and original work of two talented artists, Aslam Bashir who created the text sketches, with a pleasant blend of innocence, emotions and actions, and Danish Khan who through his title sketches and lay out design, maintained the youthful and forward looking appearance of the book without compromising on the seriousness of the contents. Bushra Khan has primarily coordinated this work. The whole outlook has been achieved after painstaking discussions and revisions; everyone's openness to ideas, suggestions and experimentation was commendable.

Conclusion

The idea behind this book is to create awareness among all caregivers, especially ECD practitioners, that child development is not in itself an end, but merely a means to community development. Thus by creating a conducive environment for children, they can contribute in human development. It requires commitment and conscientiousness to establish successful integrated ECD community-based programmes with community participation.

By no means is this text the last word on ECD; rather, it is only the development of the basic conceptual framework and guidelines for ECD-related initiatives in a developing country set-up.

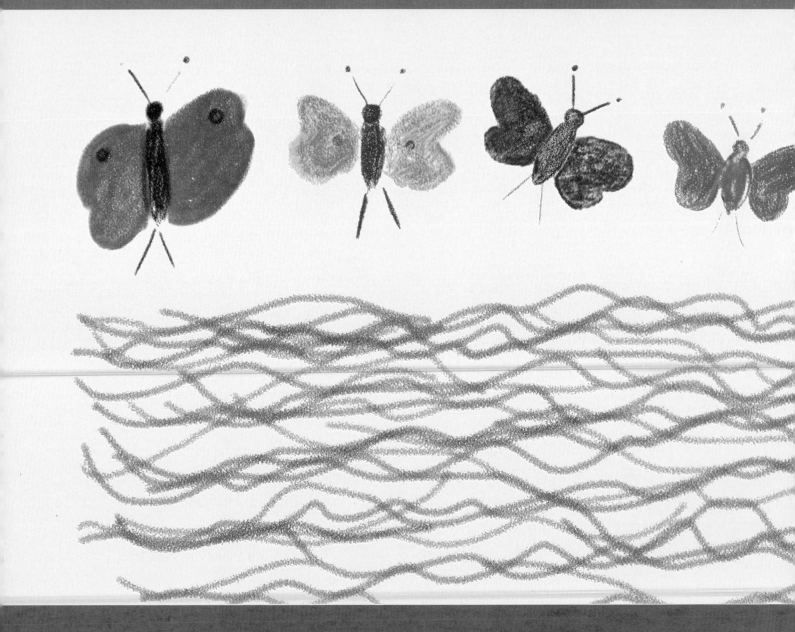

"*When the first baby laughed for the first time, the laugh broke into a thousand pieces and they all went skipping about, and that was the beginning of fairies. And now when every new baby is born its first laugh becomes a fairy. So there ought to be one fairy for every boy or girl.*"

-James Matthew Barrie

Artist:
Naushaba
Age: 6 years

Core

Concepts

Fundamentals of Child Development

Social Environment

fUNDAMENTALS OF

CHILD DEVELOPMENT

*R*ashida and Bano are sitting in a room, chatting, as a cute 16 month old Uba walks into the room towards his mother, Bano. Rashida is surprised to see that Uba has started walking without support and she greets him with affection, then starts sharing experiences with Bano about her three years old daughter, who is really a helpful child; and helps her in doing small household chores. The two friends share experiences of their children's rapid development with time. They reflect on how people change over the course of a life span.

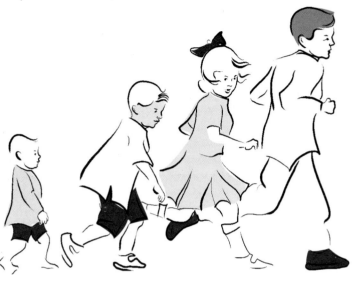

Development refers to the changes that take place in everyone's lives: in bodies, in personalities, way of thinking, feeling, behaviour and relationships and in the roles they play during the different periods of their lives. The study of Human Development encompasses virtually all these changes; the way people grow and develop, the way they learn to coordinate motor actions, and the way their personalities are formed. This growth also affects the way they think, express their emotions and respond to the special demands of their culture (1).

The process of change applies to physical, behavioural and psychological functioning.
- In the first few weeks following conception, cells are undifferentiated, as they perform no specialized function.
- A few weeks later, some cells transform into skeletal cells, some into digestive cells, others into circulatory cells and so on.
- In just the first year of life, the gross reflexive motor actions of a newborn change to more complex, specialized, and voluntary patterns of behaviour.
- In the preschooler, notions of right and wrong begin as very simple, general beliefs that develop into highly complex, individualized conceptions found among most adults.

The hierarchic integration of the changes explains the way in which differentiated parts and functions of individuals become increasingly coordinated into organized systems during development. The individual motor responses of the young infant gradually integrate into action that is more complex; for example, the coordinated motor systems eventually result in walking.

Human development is the process by which individuals; families, social groups and populations generally progress towards achieving their potential level of physical, mental, social and economic health and well-being. In human beings physical, emotional, social, cognitive development and growth occurs throughout life. Based on these changes, human development is divided into numerous phases from the time of conception until death.

Phases of Human Development

The life span of human development is usually divided into three major developmental periods: child, adolescent and adult development; each major developmental period is further divided into various sub-stages of development (2):

Child development

Prenatal period: conception through birth
Infancy: the first two years
Early childhood: 3 to 5 years
Middle childhood: 6 to 11 years

Adolescent development

Early adolescence: 12 to 14 years
Late adolescence: 15 to 19 years

Adult development

Early adulthood: 20s and 30s
Middle adulthood: 40s and 50
Late adulthood: 60 and over

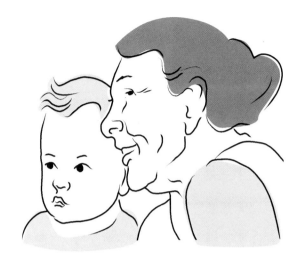

A child's developmental capabilities and needs for his or her nurturance are considerably different from any succeeding phases of human life.

All these age ranges are somewhat subjective, in that all ages for the beginning and end of the period are only approximate, and that individual people's lives are not marked off so precisely, because there is considerable variation in the development and growth of any one individual and another.

Prenatal period (conception through birth)

This includes the developmental process from conception through birth, which spans approximately nine months. During this period, basic body structure and organs are formed. Both heredity and environmental factors influence development. During the early months, the foetus is more vulnerable to negative environmental influences than during any other period of growth.

> ***CARING PRINCIPALS***
> *The prenatal period requires physical, medical and social care to achieve positive outcomes of pregnancy for the mother and her baby.*
> - *Place: Comfortable home environment and appropriately equipped health facility for safe delivery.*
> - *Persons: Family members for psychosocial support, and appropriately trained health personnel for antenatal care and delivery.*
> - *Possessions: Balanced, frequent and increased diet, in comparison to routine diet, and safe delivery kit.*

"In every child who is born, under no matter what circumstances, and of no matter what parents, the potentiality of the human race is born again: and in him, too, once more, and of each of us, our terrific responsibility toward human life."
-James Agee

Early Childhood (Birth to six years)

Infancy (The first year)

This phase from birth to 24 months is a period of tremendous changes. It is the time of extreme dependence on adults. The period, during which the processes of many psychological activities begin, mainly including language, symbolic thought, and social learning, through the child's ability to form attachments to family members and other caregivers. Infants grow in motor ability and coordination, develop sensory skills and learn to trust or distrust, and to express or withhold love and affection. They learn to express basic feelings and emotions and develop some sense of self and independence; in all these, the environment plays a vital role.

CARING PRINCIPLES
Infants are completely dependent on others, with limited prior knowledge and experience, but with eagerness to learn. Growth and development are most rapid during infancy.
- *Place: Predictable and peaceful environment*
- *Persons: Accessibility of primary caregiver with capacity to respond contingently and appropriately to the infant's needs of feeding, sleeping, clothing, hygiene and one to one interactions.*
- *Possessions: Familiar and clean meal area, sleeping space and coloured cuddly toys. Breastfeeding and age appropriate vaccination for the child Weaning diet, with gradual exposure to a large variety of food.*

Toddlerhood (1 to 5 years)

This is also referred to as the 'preschool age' or 'the preschool years'. Children continue their rapid physical, cognitive and linguistic growth. They are better able for care for themselves; begin to develop a concept of self and of gender identities and role; they become interested in playing with other children. The quality of parent-child relationships is important in the socialization process that is taking place. During this time, young children develop school readiness skills e.g. following instructions and identifying letters, and they spend many hours in play with peers.

In the literature, especially regarding ECD programming, the age groups in this period vary, and usually range from three to seven years. In this context, the book considers on average the first six years of life as the period of early child development for all discussion purposes.

> *A boy becomes an adult three years before his parents think he does, and about two years after he thinks he does.*
> -Lewis B. Hershey

CARING PRINCIPLES
Early childhood behaviour and development has a propensity to vary and move back and forth from time to time; language, reasoning and curiosity are rapidly acquired during toddlerhood.
- *Place: Safe but challenging environment to provide opportunities and resources to explore, as well as to keep pace with growth and development.*
- *Persons: Caregivers have continuous interaction and acceptance of the developmental swings of the child.*
- *Possessions: Play materials of various forms and texture, non-restricting clothing, frequent and small proportions of regular meals.*

Middle childhood (6 to 11 years)

This phase normally corresponds to the elementary school years. Children make significant advances in their ability to read; write, do arithmetic, understand their world, and think logically. Achievement becomes vitally important, as does successful adjustment with parents. Both psychosocial and moral development proceeds at a rapid rate. The quality of family relationships continues to exert a major influence on emotional and social adjustment.

CARING PRINCIPLES
Middle childhood has a remarkable capacity for memory, language, inquiry and social skills. For most children, it is also a phase of transition from home based to school based environment.
- *Place: Safe but challenging environment to provide opportunities and resources to explore, as well as to keep pace with growth and development.*
- *Persons: Multiple caregivers and peers at home and school, able to provide the opportunities of social interactions and moral reasoning.*
- *Possessions: Suitable educational materials, and a well balanced diet to meet the needs of the rapidly growing body.*

Early adolescence (12 to 14 years)

Adolescence is the period of transition between childhood and adulthood. During early adolescence, many physical changes occur that influence young peoples' lives; cognitive changes that allow them to engage in abstract thought means that their intellectual horizon can expand to include the world of possibilities. Adolescents seek greater independence from parents; they also want increased contact and a closer sense of belonging and companionship with peers.

Late adolescence (15 to 19 years)

The formation of positive identity is an important psychosocial task. The older adolescents begin to make career choices; the majority seek to complete their education, and enter the world of work.

Early adulthood (20s to 30s)

Achieving intimacy, making career choices, attaining vocational success are important challenges of early adulthood, and many decisions made during this period set the stage for later life.

Middle adulthood (40s and 50s)

During this phase, many people begin to feel a time squeeze as their biological clocks tick away. This stimulates a midlife crisis in some, during which they re-examine many facets of their lives. Many people achieve maximum personal and social responsibilities and vocational success during this period. However, adjustments need to be made to changing bodies, changing emotional, social, and job situations.

Late adulthood (60 and over)

This is the phase of adjustment particularly to changing physical, personal and social situation and relationships. Increasing attention to health care is needed to maintain vigour and well-being. The persistence of verbal skills allows some to continue to grow in knowledge and cognitive skills. Relationships with adult children, grandchildren and other relatives take on a new meaning for them at this phase of development.

All these developmental changes are the result of physical, mental and socio- emotional processes. These processes are interwoven as an individual develops, and the interplay of these processes produces the periods of human life span (3).

Our focus is on child development and within child development, infancy and early childhood are our prime phases of interest.

Adolescence is a tough time for parent and child alike. It is a time between: between childhood and maturity, between parental protection and personal responsibility, between life stage- managed by grown-ups and life privately held.
-Anna Quindlen

When I was a boy of fourteen, my father was so ignorant I could hardly stand to have the old man around. But when I got to be twenty-one, I was astonished at how much he had learned in seven years.
-Mark Twain

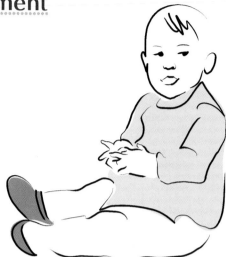

Domains of Child Development

The field of child development has been transformed into a specialized scientific discipline, and is devoted to the understanding of all aspects of human constancy and changes from conception through adolescence. Originally, its focus was on describing behaviour, so that age norms for growth and development could be derived. Recent developments in this field have integrated the patterns of development, such as understanding how children learn to speak into its focus. More emphasis is placed on the roles played by the child's surrounding environment and his/her own experiences. The discipline of child development has the following objectives in relation to the various changes occurring in a child with the passage of time:

- When these changes occur
- Under what conditions these changes occur
- How these changes influence the child's behaviour
- Whether or not these changes can be predicted

These are the domains, which encompass holistic growth and development of the child:
- Physical growth
- Mental development
- Emotional development
- Social development

Physical Growth

The extensive changes in babies' motor behaviour and cognitive abilities that occur between the ages of 2 months and 1 year depend on changes in their body proportions, muscles, bones, and brain structures (4). During the second and third years of life, children continue to grow rapidly, but the rate of their growth is considerably slower than that in the first year.

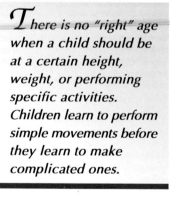

There is no "right" age when a child should be at a certain height, weight, or performing specific activities. Children learn to perform simple movements before they learn to make complicated ones.

a) Size and Shape

Most healthy babies triple in weight and grow approximately 10 inches during the first year. The rate of physical growth is greatest in the first few months after birth; it then gradually tapers off through the rest of infancy and childhood (5).

Increase in height and weight are accompanied by changes in body proportions. At birth, the head is 70 per cent of its adult size and accounts for about 25 per cent of the body's total length. At one year of age, the head accounts

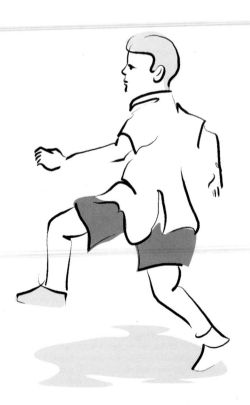

for 20 pe rcent of the body's length (6). Changes in body proportions continue to take place until about 12 months of age, making it easier for the child to balance on two legs, and begin to walk.

b) Muscle and Bone

As the child grows, bones and muscles are needed to support the increasing bulk and mobility, and they undergo corresponding growth. Most of a newborn's bones are relatively soft, and they harden gradually as minerals are deposited in them, especially during the initial months after birth. The bones in the hand and wrist are among the first to ossify (7). They harden by the end of the first year, making it easier for a baby to grasp objects, pick them up, and play with them. In infancy, increase in muscle mass is closely associated with the development of the baby's ability to stand alone and walk .

c) Brain growth

The brain develops very rapidly during this phase of development. At birth, an infant's brain weighs only about 25 percent of a mature brain. With time, the brain size increases and the brain of the two-year old child weighs 75 percent of an adult brain (8). Similarly a remarkable change happens in height and weight during this phase of development, by the end of the first year the infant's length is 50 per cent greater than it was at birth and by 2 years of age it is 75 per cent greater. Weight shows similar dramatic gains. Birth weight doubles, triples and quadruples at 5 months, 1 year and 2 years of age respectively (9). Therefore, during the first two years, these changes are rapid and faster than they will be at any time after birth.

Mental Development

Since this is the phase when the brain and neural connections develop rapidly, mental abilities of the child such as psychomotor, memory, language, thinking, reasoning, problem solving and curiosity also develop to a great extent. It is the time when a child, by using his or her five senses, i.e. touch, hearing, smell, vision

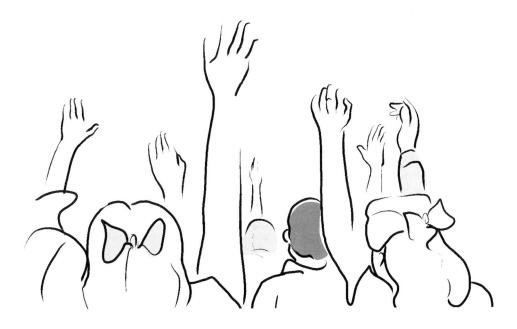

I wish I could travel by the road that crosses the baby's mind where reason makes kites of her laws and flies them.
                        -Rabindranath Tagore

Emotional Literacy means being able to recognise what you are feeling, so that it doesn't interfere with thinking. It becomes another dimension to draw upon when making decisions or encountering situations.
                        -Susie Orbach

and taste, explores the world around.

With the passage of time the coordination of mind and body, reasoning and problem solving abilities get better and better; these changes are depicted through actions, or initially, only through non verbal communication, sounds, intonations, words, and then with complete sentences. These functional abilities lay the foundation for the later mental development of the child.

Emotional Development

Emotion is a feeling-subjective sensation with observable manifestations. Emotional development refers to the development of attachment, trust, security, love, and affection, and a variety of emotions and feelings. In others words we can say that emotional development is the process by which infants and children begin to have the capacity to experience, express and interpret emotions (10).

Emotion deals with the expression and comprehension of feelings. A child initially expresses his or her emotions like happiness, anger, sadness etc. through facial expression and with time, develops the ability to comprehend the emotions of others too, which in turn affects social interaction with others.

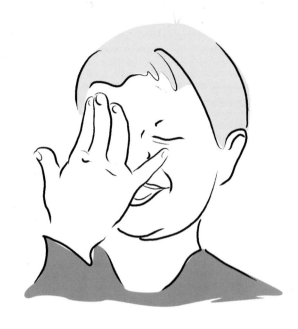

> *We know too much and feel too little. At least, we feel too little of those creative emotions from which a good life springs.*
> *-Bertrand Russell*

In addition to this, all infants and children need to form a secure emotional attachment to someone, a mother, father, other family member or a substitute caregiver (11). To feel emotionally secure, children need a warm, loving, and stable relationship with a responsive adult on whom they can depend (12). The formation of such attachments is vitally important to children's total development (13). Therefore, emotional development of children is concerned with the development of their feelings, and the expression of these feelings in relation to themselves, their parents, peers, other people and even everything in the world. Emotional development is extremely important because emotion plays an adaptive function to insure survival: for instance, feeling fear may save the child's life. They are also the means of communication; important factors in social relationship, and powerful motivators of behaviour which play a vital role in moral development.

Social Development

Children do not develop in a vacuum. They develop in the context of their family, neighbourhood, community, country and the world. In this context, children are influenced by parents, siblings, other relatives, peers, school, and groups of which they are a part. The media, community and culture in which they grow up and even the events going on in the world influence them. They are partly the product of social influences, which affect their social development.

Therefore, social development is the process

> *When the music changes, so does the dance.*
> *-African Proverb*

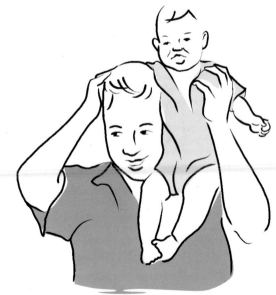

of child development based on the interaction of the individual and group through which he or she is accustomed and influenced with the societal norms and values.

Social development deals with the socialization process, i.e. the process by which persons learn the ways of society and groups so that they can function within it or them (14). Children are usually taught the ways and values of their society through contact with already socialized individuals, initially the family, which affects the social interactions of the child; this in turn affects social development. Eventually the child learns to be independent of parents by making friendships and cooperating with others.

Chart of milestones of a child from 0 to 6 is given as **Appendix I.**

Factors Affecting Child Development

Child development occurs in a holistic fashion, not in isolation. All domains of child development such as Physical growth, Mental, Social, and Emotional development are interdependent and determined by genetic potential, nutrition and health; sensory perception, social interactions and learning through exploration and experiences. It is noteworthy that all the later learning in the life of the child depends on the former growth and development by following a sequence, but the attainment of all these functional abilities could vary from individual to individual.

During the phase of infancy and early childhood, there could be numerous factors that can affect the child's development. A detailed discussion is given throughout the text; however, it can be summarized as:

Health and Nutrition

Health of the child greatly depends on the nutrition provided (15), which in turn affects his or her physical and psychological growth. Suboptimal nutrition during sensitive stages in early brain development may have long-term effects on cognitive function (16). The effect of malnutrition on the child's physical and cognitive development is as follows:

- Delayed physical growth and motor skills
- Frequent illness
- Lethargy and withdrawal
- Minimal exploration of the environment
- Brain damage
- Delayed intellectual development
- Poor cognitive development
- Greater degree of behavioural problems and deficient social skills
- Decreased attention, deficient learning, and lower educational achievement

Caregiver's attitude towards the child

The important caregivers in the lives of children seem to serve as a source of nurturance and affection that gives the youngsters confidence to explore the world and become more independent.

The caregivers who make sensible demands for maturity and have age appropriate expectations of growth, development and behaviour, enforce them by providing children with appropriate opportunities and by setting limits. At the same time, they express warmth and affection, listen patiently to their children's point of view, and encourage their participation in family decision making as they grow in age. With these considerations of a caregiver's behaviour, children develop with a lively and happy mood, self confident

Child learning takes place by linking previous experiences with current environment. Therefore, approach, potentials and expectations shaped during early childhood continue to affect learning during subsequent phases of life.

Effects of poor nutritional practices can be changed during childhood by means of targeted education and supportive interventions, resulting in improved children's health, growth rates and nutrition.

Caregiver's attention and quality time facilitates exploration by, and curiosity in the child.

Any activity becomes creative when the doer cares about doing it right, or better.
-John Updike

in their mastery of new tasks and self–controlled in their ability to resist engaging in disruptive behaviour (17).

Childcare: the behaviour and practices of caregivers are to provide
- Food
- Health care
- Sensory stimulation and
- Emotional support

Caregiver: Essential physical and psychological needs for healthy survival, growth and development of the child met by one or more people who understand what infants and children in general need
- Mothers
- Fathers
- Siblings
- Relatives, and
- Childcare service providers (e.g. education and health personnel)

Primary caregiver: The main caregiver with a capacity to respond appropriately to the child's needs of feeding, sleeping, clothing, hygiene and one to one interactions. Primary caregivers should be persistent in their responses and realistic in their expectations and should be in conformity with caring practices of secondary caregivers.

> *H*olistic Development of the child adds force to the concept that a child's growth and development potential and experiences are dependent on the overall learning prospects in the environment.

> *A* stimulating environment is created by the concerned caregivers.

Stimulating physical and social environment

The environment has a powerful influence on the development of a child's competencies. Mental development is very much influenced by the environment, which a child explores through his or her senses. The presence or absence of stimulation can speed up or slow down the acquisition of certain behaviours.

Children's capacities can be facilitated by encouraging them to manipulate the environment through play, language and problem solving skills during the second year (18). At three months of age, infants can distinguish among most colours, and can group colours into basic categories, such as reds, blues and greens (19). Provision of stimulating and safe environment enhances the mental functioning of the child.

A child is born with some characteristics in his genes, but the environment also has great impact on the child's development. If the environment is modified according to the child's learning needs the child will learn more positively. Parents not only provide the genes for the development of the child, but as caregivers also play important roles in determining the types of environment their children will encounter.

Summary

- **Human Development** encompasses all physical, emotional, intellectual, and social changes, which occur during the entire life span, which characterize human well-being and economic productivity in society.

- **Biologically,** human development can be divided into three main phases: Childhood, Adolescence and Adulthood.

- **Early childhood development** has primarily four domains: *Physical growth, mental development, social development and emotional development.*

- **Critical factors,** which affect child development, are categorized into three: *Health and Nutrition, Caregiver's attitude towards the child and Stimulating physical and social environment.*

- **Concept of child development** is perceived as changes that occur in gradual continuum associated with age; however, although the developmental pattern of the individual child varies in speed, the sequence remains predictable for most of the time.

- **A good caregiver** should be able to appreciate the facts about variation in the child's rate of growth and development, and in his or her capacity to learn new things.

Childhood should be a journey - not a race.
-Anonymous

SOCIAL ENV

RONMENT

Sameer is a 10-month old child and has an elder sister of 8 years who plays with him. His mother tries to give full attention to her young baby. She feeds him on time and provides him a healthy diet. She also brings different colourful toys for him to play with. Every evening when the child's father returns home, they go for a walk and share stories and anecdotes.

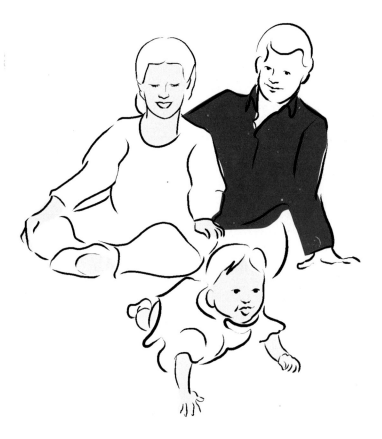

The above is a scenario of a family, which provides a good social environment to their children. The question arises here: "what is social environment?

Social Environment

Children do not develop in a vacuum; rather, they develop in the context of their family, neighbourhood, community, country and the world (1). Parents, siblings, relatives, friends, peers and other adults with whom they come in contact influence children. In addition, the media, such as radio and TV also influence children and provide sensory stimulation. Similarly, the community also influences them in terms of cultural values, laws and customs, and the list goes on. Therefore, all these factors contribute to providing sensory stimulation to the child, which affects his/her development.

Sensory Stimulation

A child gets stimulation from the environment through all five senses of hearing, touch, smell, taste and sight. The development of these senses largely depends on the sensory input a child gets from the environment. It is important to note that each sense is not isolated; rather, they work in an integrated fashion. Meaning is derived from such development, which forms part of the child's growing base of knowledge, and understanding; this determines his or her interpretation of elements encountered and experienced.

> *Home is not where you live but where they understand you.*
> *-Christian Morgenstern*

a) Auditory Sense

The sense of hearing begins before a child is born. Differentiating between sounds is a major developmental task, i.e. to exclude irrelevant sounds and attend to what is meaningful is also an important part of language development (1).

Raja listens with concentration to his mother's sounds and tries to imitate her whenever she sings a lullaby to him.

b) Tactile Sense

The sense of touch or tactile perception is the primary mode of getting stimulation from the environment. It enables the child to explore the world, and all sensations allow him to make decisions for comfort and safety. Indeed, an infant can get the feeling of security through the stimulation a caregiver provides by holding, hugging and giving other nurturing experiences. The key here is sensory input, and the type of primary stimulus in this case is tactile sensations. Early childhood experiences help children learn to identify and discriminate between tactile sensations and to make judgments about the world based on texture, temperature and pressure.

Kabir is a 2 1/2 year old child surrounded by many toys such as a soft furry teddy bear, puppets, wooden blocks and some clay toys and he is sorting out soft stuff toys from the hard ones.

c) Olfactory Sense

The olfactory sense is generally known as the sense of smell. Children's smell sensations evolve with the passage of time during early childhood, and as soon as they grow older, they can make many choices based on the smell of things; because of this, they often accept or reject experiences, settings, food, etc. because of its familiarity or unpleasantness.

Ahmed is a little child and whenever he smells even the clothes of his mother, he calms down and stops crying.

d) Gustatory Sense

The sense of taste is also called the gustatory sense. There are very few taste characteristics, which include sweet, sour, salty and bitter. Very young children do not confine their gustatory exploration to the things that one considers edible. In addition to food their tongue and mouth also experience dough, sand and toys etc., but as soon as they develop by the provision of a range of safe and satisfying taste experiences, children develop their preferences of food items which they like or dislike eating.

Sarah is a 2 1/2 year old child. When her mother puts a homemade pickle in her mouth, she spits it out at once and to change the taste, starts eating the candy, which her mother gives her.

e) Sense of Sight

Visual discrimination begins early in life (2). From infancy, a child uses visual information to make judgments and discriminate among different patterns but the ability to make fine discrimination takes many years to develop. Children normally develop visual discrimination ability in their day-to-day activities, as they play with toys, see books and materials and make decision based on what they see.

Aisha is a 3 year old child, sitting around many colourful roses that are red and yellow, and is placing the red roses at one place and the yellow at the other.

HEARING
- Musical
- Non-musical

TOUCH
- Temperature
- Pressure
- Shape/ form
- Vibration
- Texture
- Pain

SMELL
- Pleasant
- Aversive

TASTE
- Sweet
- Sour
- Saltish
- Bitter

VISION
- Light
- Colour
- Pattern
- Depth
- Texture
- Movement

All sensory stimulations that a child receives from the environment result in neural connections, which lead to the development of the brain.

"Home is the one place in all this world where hearts are sure of each other. It is the place of confidence."
-Frederick W. Robertson

As we discuss the social environment, we view the child developing within the system of relationships affected by multiple levels of the environment. This provides us an opportunity to observe closely the effects of social environment on a child in relation to the specific environmental context.

The Social Environment Context of Early Childhood Development

The social environment has a great effect on children's physical, mental, social and emotional development. The environment that plays an important role in the development of children, unfolds itself through different levels. Initially, a child's environment comprises family, parents, siblings and grandparents, then his or her social exposure widens, i.e. beyond home there is school and other neighbourhood settings in which children spend their everyday lives (3, 4, 5).

Internal Relationships: Family Interaction

The family is the child's foremost context of development. Family provides nutrition, hygiene, security, safe physical environment, opportunities to play and to explore objects; the family also introduces children to the physical world. Within the family, children acquire language, an abundance of useful information and skills, an understanding of themselves and other people, and moral and cultural values. The love, affection and security children receive from the family have long lasting effect on their further relationships in the future. It is important to note that all relationships are bi-directional, so that both adults and children affect each other's behaviour in a positive manner.

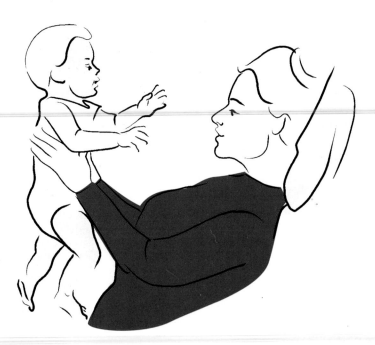

Daud's parents enjoy playing with him, because he is a very friendly and attentive child, whereas Naseem is a quite unfriendly and non-responsive child, and is often restricted by his parents.

Relationships with family members, with not only parents but also siblings and grandparents affect children's attitudes.

Quality time that parents or caregivers give to the children in talking, playing, reading and disciplining, include ways of interaction that encourage children's expanding motor, cognitive and social skills. It also establishes a strong bond between children and caregiver, and develops the trust, which the children can generalize towards others.

Obi is a 2-year-old boy watching T.V. His mother comes into the room and says, "Obi do you remember Ahmed uncle presented a beautiful toy car to you?" He replies, "Yes Ami, it is really beautiful." His mother says, "Let's play with it. I'll tell you how you can play with it; there is a key, now you turn it and put the car on the floor." Obi says happily, "Oh! It is really great." His mother looks at him affectionately. Obi's mother spends around two hours with him then she says now it is your sleeping time. Obi goes to his elder sister who tells him the story of a brave boy. Suddenly he quarrels with his sister and starts crying. Their mother comes and says "Obi what are you doing? Good boys don't behave like this". Then his sister again starts the story and he feels happy and asks many questions. Finally, he sleeps.

Siblings exert considerable influence on younger brothers and sisters. Elder siblings are nurturing when interacting with their little sisters and brothers. During play, they learn competence, cooperation, and sharing, and then learn these functions successfully in peer groups.

Grandparents can promote children's development in many ways; both directly by responding warmly to the child and indirectly, by providing parents with childrearing advice.

The learning materials that are given to the child are another source of sensory stimulation in the home environment. they help children to develop and explore their physical limits and creativity.

Reena is a 3-year-old child, enjoying her creativity, as she makes utensils with clay and water.

In like manner, the safe physical environment of the home helps a child to explore the world around him or her.

Gul was playing with his sister in the yard, when suddenly he cried and his sister called her mother. His mother found a small piece of glass that he had cut his foot with and was bleeding.

The physical environment available to the child should be clean and free from hazards. The physical hazards such as a stove in a yard, broken glass lying around, uncovered rotary fan, unprotected stairs for toddling (pre-walking) baby that could injure children. If the physical environment is not safe for children, it would be dangerous for them to play freely and could cause parents to place restrictions on their activities.

Indirect influences of family are important, and can serve as effective support for child development, or alternatively, they can undermine a child's well being. When parents' marital relationship is warm and considerate, mother and father praise and stimulate their children more and scold them less. In contrast, when a marriage is tense and hostile, parents are likely to express anger, criticise and punish. Similarly, when quarrelsome relations exist between parents and grandparents, it may adversely affect parent-child interaction. Therefore, a wide range of relationships: mother with father, parents with sibling, grandparent with parents, affect the child's development.

External Relationships: Neighbourhoods, Childcare Centres or Schools, and Play Areas

For children to develop to their best, child-rearing support must also exist in the larger environment. It

Loving a baby is a circular business, a kind of feedback loop. The more you give the more you get and the more you get the more you feel like giving.
-Penelope Leach

SAFE ENVIRONMENT
Indications of danger or abuse are promptly recognized and minimized or removed, to make children feel more secure in the environment.

encompasses connection between children's immediate settings such as home, school, neighbourhood, and childcare centre that foster children's development. Neighbourhoods play an important role in children's development. Safe physical environment of the neighbourhood, such as danger-free manholes, covered drainage and clean and straight road surfaces help the child to walk and run easily. When children play in the neighbourhood, they learn to interact and to cooperate with people. Similarly, the neighbourhood's adults play an important role; besides behaviour, language and character development, they also keep a watchful eye on the activities of children.

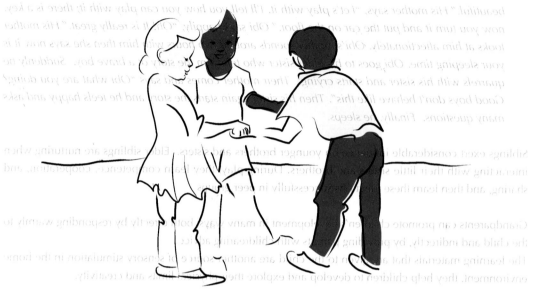

School or childcare centres provide social experiences under the guidance of trained teachers who promote enjoyable contacts and try to give opportunities in group participation and better social adjustment. However, the children's academic progress depends on not only activities that take place in the classroom, but also on their parents' involvement in their school life, and the extent to which academic learning is carried over at home. The links between home and childcare settings affect the child's development in the form of visits and exchange of information. Even availing the facility of the play area in the community helps in children development.

External relationships promote many aspects of a child's wellbeing, including self-confidence, school performance and educational aspirations. Eventually, these children will become productive members of their society.

External Services: Workplace, Community Health Services

The external services that are not directly connected with children but affect their experiences in immediate settings, may be formal organizations, such as work place or health and welfare services in the community, or social networks. For instance, affordable community health services play an important role in children's development in terms of treatment, vaccination etc. Work settings can help parents in their childrearing roles, and indirectly enhance development by offering flexible work schedules, paid maternity and sick leave.

Naveen's mother works in the fields from dawn till dusk, but can have a flexible schedule whenever Ahmed is ill.

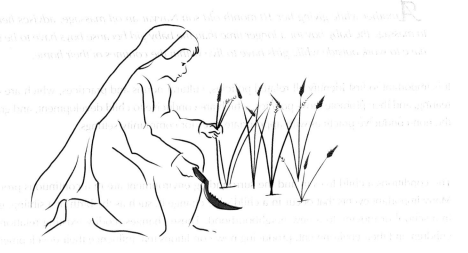

External services can be informal, such as parents' social networks, friends and relatives who provide advice, companionship, and even financial assistance. They can be a great support and source for social development of the child.

Socio-cultural & Political Context

The home environment and neighbourhoods are important in children's development; in addition; culture, political support and child-friendly policies at national level are also significant factors.

Every culture has different customs and values and has both positive and negative effects. Living together with parents and grandparents in a joint family system enhances love among them, and they can share their happiness as well as grievances. Other than this, all the members of the family look after the child; this enhances the child's development in a better way.

An angels single feather,
Also a dash of love and care,
Then mix them both together.
Add a sentiment or two,
A thoughtful wish or line,
A touch of stardust, a sunshine ray,
Its a recipe, for a Baby Girl truly fine.

-Anonymous

Children should be accepted and nurtured irrespective of their potentials and credentials.

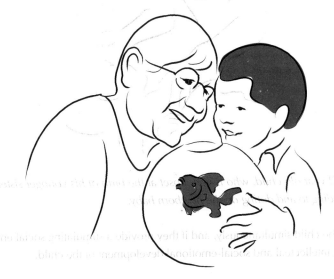

It is important to identify detrimental cultural practices for child development and conscious efforts should be made to modify them. As in most of the developing countries, there is a concept that boys should be given every opportunity for higher studies but not girls, because after marriage girls have to live within the family environment, while boys become a permanent support to their families.

A mother while giving her 10 month old son Nayyar an oil massage, advises her younger sister to massage the baby boy for a longer time than the baby girl because boys have to be stronger as they have to work outside while girls have to live within the confines of their home.

It is important to first identify all related policies, cultural norms and practices, which are related to child rearing, and then promote those policies, which are conducive to child development, and gradually replace the non-conducive practices with appropriate ones for community settings.

Significant Life Events

The conditions a child lives in and the surrounding environment are in a continuous process of change. Many important events that occur in a child's life change it, such as the birth of a sibling, getting enrolled in a school or moving to a new neighbourhood. These changes modify existing relationships between children and their environment, producing new conditions that influence their development (6).

Likewise, starting school brings a change in the child's life. Before starting, he was confined to his home but now he starts interacting with a number of people including class fellows, teachers and other people associated with school. He/she also begins formal studies.

Usually the birth of a sibling affects the child because parents and other family members give more attention to a newly born child.

> *Come out of the circle of time
> And into the circle of love.*
> -Rumi

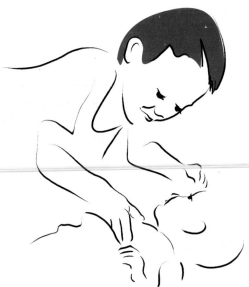

Yousaf is a 2 1/2 year old child, who is very upset at the birth of his younger sister as everyone in the family is attending to and doting on the newborn baby.

The list of considerations in this document is indicative rather than definitive. Each early childhood setting will develop its own emphases and priorities.

All these levels affect the child simultaneously, and if they provide a stimulating social environment, they lead to better physical, intellectual and social-emotional development of the child.

Consideration of Social Environment by the Caregiver

Social environment for children 0-6 years should address their physical, socio-emotional, psychological and stimulatory needs. To address the needs of growing children, conducive social environment can be categorized into the following domains. It is important to note that the concept of a child's environment is applicable to the home, day-care centre, school or any setting which the child is experiencing on a regular basis. A caregiver is any person who is looking after or taking care of a child in these settings. It could be a parent, relatives, siblings, teachers and even health personnel. Regardless of the type of caregiver, always take a critical look as a first step whenever you enter into a child related environment. The purpose of the environmental appraisal, however, is to emphasize the importance of suggestions for implementation of constructive changes in it.

The list of considerations in this document is indicative rather than definitive. Each early childhood setting will develop its own emphases and priorities.

Caregiver Involvement

The level of interest, emotion and activity that the caregiver is prepared to expend on the child represents a caregiver's reaction to the child's behaviour; in turn, the caregiver reinforces it through all means, both verbally and physically, by showing care and affection. The quality of being responsive assumes that the caregiver understands the child has needs, and responds quickly to the child.

Child Development and Behaviour Status

It is the level of human interactions, based on acceptance of less than optimum performance and behaviour from the child by the caregiver, and the avoidance of undue checks and penalties. This process also requires tolerance and readjustment of the expectation from the caregiver on regular basis. The extension of this concept is unconditional acceptance of children of different cultures, religions, and gender, in classroom and health care settings.

Order and Organization

This describes the level to which there is regularity in the schedules at home and in school, in a safe physical setting. It does not mean that the environment is firm and constant, and does not allow new avenues for exploration. This concept also extends to non-conflicting roles and behaviours of the caregivers, and communication of clear rules and their consequences by them.

Assortment of Interactions

These indicate the level of additions of new people and events in their life schedule without compromising on order and organization. It is equally applicable in the classroom setting by following the order and organization of the timetable; new related learning tasks are offered in the classrooms.

Learning Opportunities

These spell the level of age appropriate provision and authorization to manipulate play and learning materials capable of stimulating the child. These materials help the child in refinement of skills, which must be acquired during the early childhood period. Home or classroom environment should promote positive behaviour and learning for children with varied learning characteristics, as changes in an individual's behaviour arising from experience. An emphasis will be placed on manipulative materials and real-life experiences.

Significance of Social Environment

Physical Development

- An effective social environment focuses on fulfilment of the basic needs of the child such as food,

If evolution really works, how come mothers only have two hands?
-Milton Berle

If opportunity doesn't knock, build a door.
-Milton Berle

The art of progress is to preserve order amid change and to preserve change amid order.
-Alfred North Whitehead

Both interior and exterior components of the environment should be considered learning resources for the growing child.

shelter, education and healthy surroundings, which definitely prevent the child from illnesses and help in his physical development.

- Stimulating environments facilitate the psychomotor development of the child as he/she can achieve the milestones either at the appropriate age or even before the due age.
- Through stimulation more neuronal connections form, which develop the brain and as a result, the child acquires motor, cognitive and social skills.

Cognitive Development

- The child can understand the concepts of similarity and difference and learn to sort out things based on this concept.
- A stimulating environment helps to develop the reasoning ability of a child.
- The social environment improves the problem-solving abilities of a child.
- A positive social environment helps prepare the child for developing language skills and improves memory.
- Through the social environment, the child learns the cause and effect relationship on which he/she has to determine his behaviour in a social environment.
- Social environment provides the opportunities of trial and error by which a child learns in every day life.
- A stimulating environment prepares the child for better future performance in school and enhances professional skills.

Emotional Development

- Social environment determines the self-concept of the child. The nature of a child's self-concept depends on interaction with family members or other significant persons (e.g. teachers, neighbours), and the mode and contents of communication with them. Self-concept influences the child's ability to develop meaningful relationships with people and the surrounding world.
- A child who gets all due love and care develops trust, which he or she can generalize to the external world.
- A stimulating environment helps children to understand their own emotional state as well as that of others. They learn to express emotions, which in turn help them to communicate their feelings and ideas.
- A child learns social interactions so that he or she can adjust and function effectively with people.
- In a stimulating environment, children appear to be more socially skillful, more curious, independent and persistent in approaching new tasks, and more mature.

Summary

- **Social environment** comprises people, places, and things in the child's surroundings
- **Learning** primarily takes place through sensory stimulation of five senses: hearing (auditory), touch (tactile), smell (olfactory), taste (gustatory), and vision (sight).
- **The Social environment** has five critical layers: *Internal Relationships: family interaction, External Relationships: neighbourhoods, childcare centres or schools, and play areas, External Services: workplace, community health services, cultural context and significant life events.*
- **The child learns** through active exploration and interaction with the environment. A child's learning environment extends the immediate setting of the home, child related institutions and respective community status.

- **The quality of the social environment** can be evaluated by its five main contents: *Caregiver's Involvement, Child Development and Behavioural Status, Order and Organization, Assortment of Interactions and Learning Opportunities.*

- **Quality time** given by the caregiver is primarily spent with children for the purpose of talking, playing, reading and disciplining. These ways of interacting encourage the children's expanding motor, cognitive and social skills.

- **Human Interaction** enables children to make sense of places, events and people, and provides opportunities to learn by trying out their concepts with adults as well as other children.

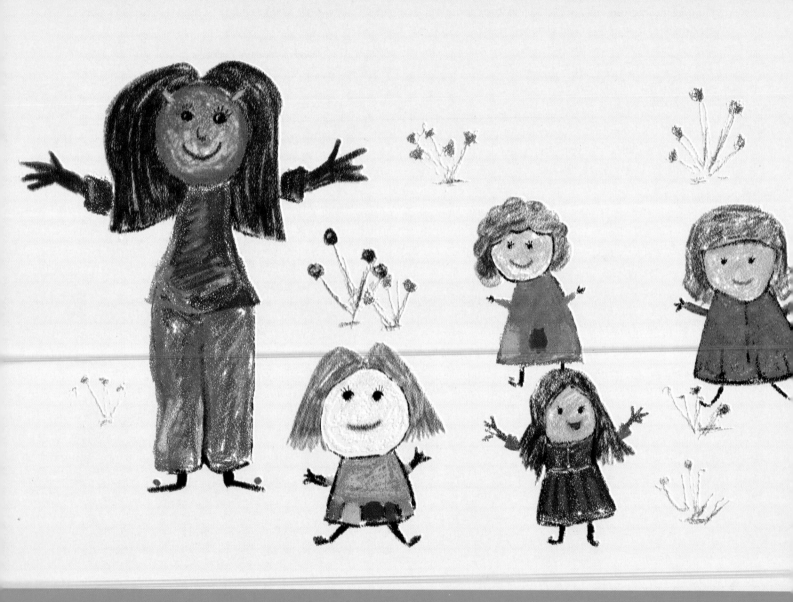

"*If you cannot teach me to fly, teach me to sing.*
-James Matthew Barrie"

Artist:
Soha
Age: 6 years

part 6

ASSESSMENT AND ADVICE

GENERAL GUIDELINES

FOR CHILD ASSESSMENT

*O*ne evening Hamida came to Shabana's house, where Shabana was playing with her son. Hamida knocked on the door and went inside, Shabana greeted her warmly;

Hamida: what's the matter, Shabana? You look worried.

Shabana: Well, my son is 12 months old and he is still not walking.

Hamida: Oh! That's really not a good sign, because my daughter started walking when she was 10 months old.

Shabana: Oh! my God is there really something wrong with my son…?

> *W*hen I approach a child, he inspires in me two sentiments; tenderness for what he is, and respect for what he may become.
> -Louis Pasteur

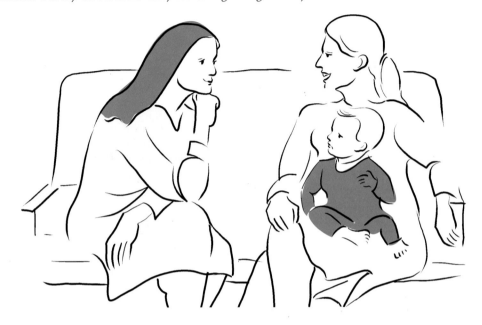

This scenario shows a worried mother whose uncertainty can be resolved by appropriate assessment. But the question arises, whether Shabana's assessment methodology is correct or not?

Child Assessment

It is the measurement of various aspects related to physical growth, child behaviour and mental processes on the basis of specific criteria.

Need for Assessment

Assessment of children is needed to know child's intellectual, psychomotor (physical), and emotional development and growth.

- *Intellectual Assessment* is needed to explore the child's ability to learn and reason; his/her capacity for knowledge and understanding
- *Psychomotor Assessment* will be required in case a mother/father complains that her child is not sitting even at the age of 9 months, or in similar cases.
- *Emotional Assessment* can be done in case a caregiver says that her child avoids people and does not interact with them, or in similar cases.
- *Growth Assessment* can be looked for when a child has not gained appropriate weight or height as compared to the children of same age group.

Therefore, assessment plays a key role in identifying problems and developing intervention strategies for children.

SCREENING
A preliminary assessment of the child for early identification of any developmental delay or growth

Precautions for Child Assessment

Before administering the assessment tool one should keep the following precautions in mind (1):

Advance Preparation for Assessment

Before starting an assessment it is extremely important to read the guidelines accompanying the assessment instrument, with special attention. This will enable the assessor to know the purpose of the test and directions for administration.

It is really helpful to memorize the exact verbal instruction because some previous familiarity with the statement to be read prevents misreading and hesitation and gives confidence and a natural manner during assessment.

Test Materials

Test materials actually comprise different objects that are required for conducting certain assessment. Therefore, it is necessary that all materials of the applied test be well organized ahead of time to avoid hassles. Sometimes the assessor realizes the absence of certain materials when he/she is half way through the assessment session.

Testing Conditions

Testing can take place at a facility or at home; the place where the assessment is going to be carried out must be spacious: it could either be a room or a courtyard in rural areas, so that the child is able to do physical tasks easily, for instance, in a psychomotor assesment if a child is asked to hop to a certain distance then space is required. Proper lighting and ventilation are also needed to facilitate the assessment session.

It usually happens that family members gather around the child at the testing place. Make sure that their presence does not affect the assessment. Family members often try to guide the child by suggesting what comes next. The assessor should tell the family members not to prompt during the assessment, otherwise the child attention would be divided and he/she may not perform according to his/her own abilities. It does happen though, that the presence of others either facilitates the child's performance or hampers it.

It is recommended that the assessment be conducted in seclusion provided that the child is comfortable with the assessor. If this is not the case, then initially it should be done in the presence of the caregiver, and as soon as rapport is built, the assessment can begin where chances of presence of others is minimal.

Physical Health of a Child

Before starting assessment, make sure that the child is not ill and does not show the explicit signs of irritability, physical and mental disability otherwise the child will not be able to respond in accordance with his/her abilities.

Physiological Need of a Child

It is important to make sure that the physiological needs of a child have been met, i.e. the child has eaten and had a sound sleep. If these needs are not fulfilled, the child will not be able to perform to optimal abilities.

Rapport

The term rapport refers to familiarity and friendliness with a person. To obtain the child's optimal performance,

> *No one tests the depth of a river with both feet.*
> -African Proverb

> *Adults should understand the progression and variations of children's development and should provide time for gradual growth of independent skills.*

the assessor must establish rapport with him/ her (2, 3). As we are working with children aged between 0 to 6 years, it would be helpful to focus on rapport building according to their age:

CAUTION
- *A child who shies away on being observed or tested must not be observed, until rapport is established*
- *A child who becomes anxious must be comforted;*
- *Any threat to the child's self-esteem must be avoided.*

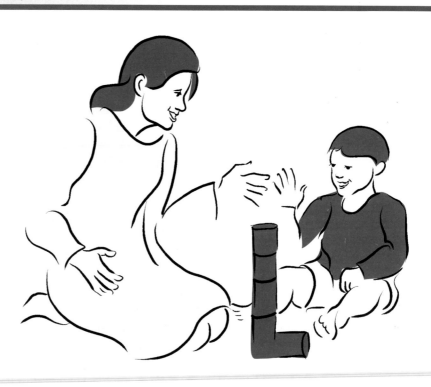

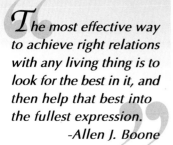

The most effective way to achieve right relations with any living thing is to look for the best in it, and then help that best into the fullest expression.
-Allen J. Boone

Building rapport with infants (0 to 1 $^{1}/2$ years)
- It is better to approach infants in an unhurried and friendly manner. Often the best way is to focus the initial attention on the infant's primary caregiver, e.g. mother, this helps the child to observe the interaction between assessor and the caregiver and facilitates the infant's feeling of comfort with the assessor and the assessment session.

- At the beginning of the session, look towards and smile at the infant and if he /she responds or attempts to interact with the assessor then respond to him/ her in a calm and friendly manner.

Praise your children and they will blossom.

- It is advisable not to take the infant from the caregiver's arms and start assessment because this behaviour of the assessor might irritate the child and consequently affect the assessment results.

- It is possible that infants as young as 9 months show anxiety in the presence of a stranger; this is the child's expression of fear in response to an unfamiliar adult, so it is better to allow the infant to sit in the caregiver's lap while being assessed.

Building rapport with toddlers (1 $^{1}/2$ to 2 $^{1}/2$)
- Like an infant, a child of this age group may show anxiety towards a stranger: to overcome that, allow the child to become familiar with the assessor; and ask for the caregiver's assistance, when needed.

- Try to talk to and encourage the child, using language whenever possible rather then focusing on just gestures. The assessor can start a conversation by praising, which can bridge the gap between assessor and the child. The assessor must maintain friendly interaction with the child.

"What a nice colour of your suit, who bought it?"
"The ball is fun to play with. Would you like to play with me?"

Building rapport with preschoolers (2^1/2 to 3 years)

- To gain the cooperation of a child of this age group requires full attention to the child. Preschoolers are likely to be initially shy in performing tasks even if the caregiver is present, therefore, try to start a conversation about the child's interest or activities.

- With a shy child it is better to start with active tasks that do not require verbal responses, because by the time, the child responds, he/she will start speaking.

- It is advisable that the assessor be sensitive to a child who uses "I cannot" or "I don't" as a way of indicating fatigue or boredom with the assessment procedure. In this case, the assessor should immediately stop the activity and try to participate in whatever is the primary interest of the child, so that the child's attention in the assessment is revived.

Building rapport with children aged between 3 to 6 years:

- Like preschoolers children of this age group could be shy or reluctant to interact with the assessor. Therefore it would be better if the assessor starts a conversation with the caregiver and during that breaks the ice with the child while talking about any usual thing, like in which class he/she is studying in, or what games he/she likes to play.

- Since children of this age range can communicate well through language, it would be good if the assessor, rather than starting assessment abruptly, explains in very simple words about the item of the assessment to the child so that he/she becomes comfortable with the assessment session.

Do you like to colour? I have blocks of different colours, from which you can sort out each colour.

- Sometimes it so happens that children seem very uncomfortable with the presence of a stranger, so it is helpful if the assessor is innovative, and lets the child become involved in activities similar to those required in the assessment in a non directional way. As soon as the child gets familiar with the assessor, proceed to the assessment.

Rapport with the caregiver

Child assessment especially at community level is not possible without establishing rapport with the caregiver. This person is in close contact with the child, and the child himself feels secure and comfortable with him/her. It is important to take the consent of the caregiver regarding child assessment and let him/her know about the purpose of the assessment.

As soon as the caregiver becomes clear about the purpose and significance of the assessment, he/she starts playing a crucial role in building rapport between the child and the assessor that helps to run the assessment procedure smoothly.

You can't shake hands with a clenched fist.
-Indira Gandhi

Conceptual understanding of a child's nature

Temperament

Every child is born with a set of unique features which determine the individual variations in emotional self regulation, i.e., Quality and intensity of emotional reaction (4, 5, 6). Temperament has the following salient characteristics:

- **Activity level:** Predisposition of vigour and self-motivation as compared to passive and immobile.
- **Approach:** Predisposition of moving eagerly towards new people, objects or experiences. It is an indication of positive emotionality.
- **Irritability:** Predisposition of moving angrily away from or towards new people, objects or experiences. It is an indication of negative emotionality.
- **Inhibition and anxiety:** Predisposition of responding with fear or nervousness towards new people, objects or experiences
- **Task persistence:** Predisposition of maintaining concentration and effort for a task

Temperament of children can be broadly categorised as;

Easy child: Temperament is characterized by high levels of
- Activity level
- Approach
- Task persistence

Low levels of
- Irritability
- Inhibition and anxiety

The child rapidly begins regular routines in infancy, is generally happy, and adapts easily to new experiences.

Slow to warm up child: Temperament is characterized by high levels of
- Inhibition and anxiety
- Approach
- Task persistence

Low levels of
- Activity level
- Irritability

Child shows mild, low-key reactions to environmental stimuli, is passive in mood and adjusts slowly to new experiences.

Difficult child:

Temperament is characterized by high levels of
- Activity level
- Irritability

Low levels of
- Inhibition and anxiety

- Task persistence
- Approach

Child is irregular in daily routines, is slow to accept new experiences, and tends to react negatively and intensely with anger.

	Easy Child	Slow to warm up Child	Difficult Child
Activity Level	High	Low	High
Approach	High	High	Low
Task persistence	High	High	Low
Inhibition and Anxiety	Low	High	Low
Irritability	Low	Low	High

High Level ▮
Low Level

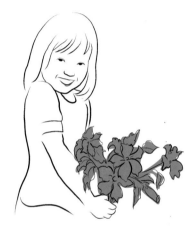

Easy children are quite welcoming to new experiences and less hesitant to initiate any task without the fear of failure. Building rapport and doing the assessment in a playful manner would be a pleasant experience for them.

Slow to warm up children sometimes take time to exhibit the interest in the process and usually need the caregiver's support and encouragement to initiate the task required for the testing. As soon as rapport with the assessor establishes child gradually starts accepting the challenges of the assessment procedure and cooperate with the assessor.

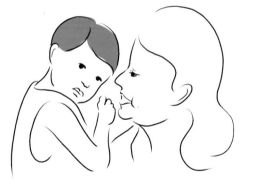

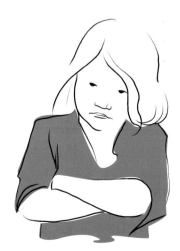

Difficult children are tough but not impossible to work with. They are quite resistant in accepting new situations, experiences and persons, and sometimes react in an extremely negative fashion.

> *Consideration of temperament helps run a smooth child assessment procedure.*

> *All children are artists. The problem is how to remain an artist once he grows up.*
> *-Pablo Picasso*

- During assessment initial focus is on rapport building with the caregiver: continue talking with the caregiver so that the child becomes familiar with the assessor.
- Assessment should begin with observation or with tasks which do not need the interference or instruction of the assessor so that the child feels free to adjust to the environment.
- By the time the child settles into the new situation, and then with the help of the caregiver gradually interacts with the assessor, the latter should initiate assessment based on instructions in a playful manner.

It is important to keep in mind that the assessor constantly encourages and accepts the child's interest level in assessment. Sensitivity to the mood swings of this child is important in order to avoid any negative response which can affect the later assessment procedure.

Who can assess:

Child assessment could be in a home based or facility based setting. Minimal criteria for the assessor and outcome of the assessment vary in each setting.

1. Household based assessment (Community):

Community based workers with preliminary academic credentials can be formally trained to conduct home based assessments. The purpose of this assessment would be

- To assess and maintain the record of developmental status at periodic intervals
- To suggest measures to enhance growth and development of the child
- To screen the children for any developmental delays
- To refer the developmentally delayed children to the facility for further evaluation

2. Facility based assessments:

A trained professional with relevant academic credentials is a prerequisite to conduct Facility based assessments. The purpose of this assessment would be

- To confirm the diagnosis of the children for any developmental delays
- to suggest any remedial measures to correct the developmental delay

STEPWISE CONSIDERATION TO INITIATE A CHILD'S ASSESSMENT
- *Start a conversation with the caregiver, for instance by letting him/her know the purpose of the study.*
- *As soon as rapport with the caregiver is built, the child would start feeling comfortable in the assessor's presence.*
- *Now start getting the child's attention by smiling at him/her.*
- *Call out the child's name and when the child responds, gradually interact with him/her.*
- *Now the assessor can start praising his toys and keep asking, for example, who has bought this toy? How does it work? How do we play with it? And so on.*
- *Now the assessor can ask the child if he/she would like to play with him (the assessor). Assessor can use the toy which is the part of assessment tool, to gain the child's attention and start playing with him.*
- *As soon as the assessor realizes that the child has become familiar with him/her the assessment process can gradually be started.*
- *Try to standardize the duration of the process.*

Try to complete the assessment in a playful manner in order to maintain rapport with the child.

Summary

- **Child Assessment** is the process of the measurement of various aspects related to physical growth, child behaviour and mental abilities on the basis of specific criteria.

- **Assessment of children** is needed in order to know their intellectual, psychomotor (physical), and emotional development and growth.

- **Precautions for Child Assessment** includes advance preparation for assessment especially test materials and testing conditions, consideration for physical health, physiological needs of a child, rapport building with child and caregiver.

- **Rapport** refers to familiarity and friendliness with a child.

- **Personality** is a distinctive and in an overall manner relatively stable patterns of each child of reacting to and interacting with others.

- **Temperament** is the emotional foundation of personality, partially determined by genetics.

NUTRITION, GROWTH

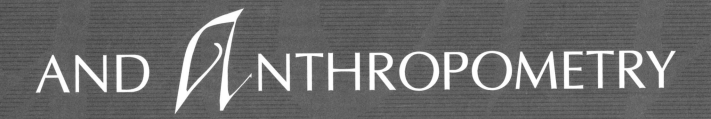

AND ANTHROPOMETRY

It is a pleasant March morning in a remote village of district Dadu. A group of children are playing in the open field adjacent to the rice crop. They are of more or less the same age, that is, three years. They are very happy, active and alert. Their hair and eyes look shiny, and the skin is smooth in spite of the complexion differences. Close to these children there is another child of the same age, sitting quietly. He looks very weak and lethargic; his height is also less than that of the other children. He has very fine thin hair, protruded abdomen and very dry skin. He does not seem to be at all interested in the game being played by the other children.

> *To keep the body in good health is a duty.... otherwise we shall not be able to keep our mind strong and clear.*
>
> *-Buddha*

NUTRITION:
Knowledge of composition of nutrients of food and their effects on health.

CALORIE: *A unit of measure of the amount of energy supplied by food.*

NUTRIENTS:
Chemical substances found in foods that are used by the body for growth and health.
The six categories of nutrients are
- *Carbohydrates*
- *Proteins*
- *Fats*
- *Vitamins*
- *Minerals*
- *Water*

Although the children are residents of the same area, and belong to the same age group and socioeconomic status, what do you think could be the reason for these differences?

Nutrition, Growth & Development

Nutrition is the science by which we take in and use food for the maintenance of life, growth, organ and tissue functioning and production of energy (1). Nutrition can be defined as the science of food and its nutrients, and their relation to health (2).

- Good nutrition is essential to the health and well-being of individuals, whether a child, an adult or an elderly person. Nutrition is not only important from the viewpoint of an individual, but also for the entire population. In this chapter, we will consider measurements of the physical dimensions of the body as a means of assessing nutritional status.

Nutrients

It is important to distinguish between diet and nutrients. Diet is the source of nutrients. Nutrients are the nourishing substances in food that are essential for the growth and development of the child leading to adulthood, and for the maintenance of body functions throughout life. The six main categories of nutrients in diet include (3, 4, 5): **(See Appendix II)**

1. Carbohydrates

These are the primary sources for energy to the body. They include starches, sugars, fruits (e.g. apple, banana, etc.) and vegetables (e.g. potatoes, etc.).

2. Proteins;

Their main function is to build tissues. Proteins ensure growth and maintenance of a strong body structure. Proteins can be derived from animal sources (e.g. milk, meat, eggs, etc.) and plant sources (e.g. legumes and lentils, etc.).

3. Fats

Fats act as a storage form of heat and energy for the body. They protect the body against mechanical injury by providing padding and support to the body organs. Fats also act as insulators against rapid body temperature changes. The animal sources of fats include butter, milk, egg, meat, etc., and vegetable sources include vegetable oil and ghee.

4. Vitamins

These are the substances which help to release the energy trapped in carbohydrates, fats, and proteins. Deficiency of any vitamin can lead to various diseases. Two major categories of vitamins include:

a)   Fat soluble vitamins, namely A (found in milk, butter, egg, carrot, spinach), D (found in milk, butter, egg, oil, ghee, and exposure of skin to sunlight), E (found in green leafy vegetables, cereals and pulses) and K (found in cabbage, milk, soya bean and eggs etc.).

b)   Water soluble vitamins include Vitamin B complex (found in liver, meat, egg, milk, legumes, wheat etc) and C (found in uncooked green leafy vegetables, oranges, lemon, guava, tomatoes etc).

5. Minerals

Minerals are essential for maintaining the body in a healthy state. They are utilized in every chemical and physical reaction in the body. Calcium is found in milk, leafy vegetables and soya beans; Phosphorus is present in eggs, milk, meat, cereals and soya bean etc. and Iron in liver, meat, green leafy vegetables etc. Deficiency of any particular mineral can result in various diseases. Calcium and phosphorus are necessary for the formation of bones and teeth. Similarly iron is needed for the formation of blood.

6. Water

It functions as a regulatory agent. It is the fundamental agent of life, which is required for all processes involved in the digestion and absorption of food in the body.

Note: carbohydrates, proteins and fats form the major components of diet, whereas vitamins and minerals are needed in smaller amounts.

MINERALS:
There are 15 essential minerals required in the diet.
- *Deficiency diseases occur when too little of any of these is provided to the body*
- *Toxicity reactions occur when too much is provided.*

ECD REINFORCEMENTS
Nutrition
Eating five or more servings of fruits and vegetables is a good way of getting enough vitamins in the diet each day.

WATER IN THE BODY
- *Regulates body temperature*
- *Transports nutrients*
- *Removes waste products*
- *Assists in energy formation*

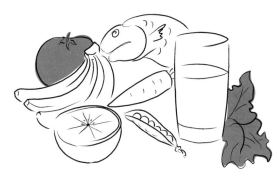

Adequate nutrition is required for the entire life of an individual, but it is extremely important during the early years of life, as this period is critical from the growth and development perspective. Moreover, this is the period in which both these phenomena occur most rapidly.

Nutrition has a significant role in the maintenance of health, promotion of growth and provision of resistance to disease. Early nutrition in foetal life and childhood has both short and long term consequences in later life (6).

Proper Nutrition

It affects brain development, 70% of which occurs in utero; the final stages occur within 18-24 months of birth. Children with proper early nutrition have optimum brain development, which results in their better intellectual and educational performance. Proper nutrition leads to appropriate growth and increased muscle mass which results in better immunity against diseases and achievement of body size. These can predict work performance and capacity in the long run. Studies reveal that food supplementation during early childhood results in taller adults with greater lean body mass and work capacity (7).

Malnutrition

It is a continuous threat to the health of children in developing countries. A child who is malnourished lags far behind in terms of physical and mental growth than his/her properly nourished colleagues. This undernourished status and halted growth is indicated primarily by subnormal values on physical measurements.

> *MALNUTRITION:*
> *Poor nutrition resulting from an excess or lack of calories or nutrients. Malnutrition early in life has long-term effects on mental and physical development.*
> *An improvement in nutritional status in children reduces rates of:*
>
> | Immediate | Long term |
> |---|---|
> | • *Congenital abnormalities* | •• *Overweight* |
> | • *Growth retardation* | •• *Hypertension, heart disease and stroke* |
> | • *Mental retardation* | •• *Diabetes* |
> | • *Iron deficiency* | •• *Osteoporosis* |
> | • *Baby bottle tooth decay* | •• *Cancer* |
> | • *Food allergy* | |

Malnutrition and mental performance

Like physical growth, mental development too is influenced by diet. Since the major part of brain growth occurs during pregnancy and the initial years of life, malnutrition during that period can have profound negative effects on mental development. Adverse mental effects of early malnutrition include poor memory, low intelligence, short attention span etc (8).

> *HEALTHY DIET*
> *is characterized by balance, adequacy and variety.*
> * *Balanced diet: A diet that provides neither too much nor too little from all the categories of nutrients.*
> * *Adequate diet: A diet consisting of foods that together supply sufficient protein, vitamins, and minerals and as many calories as necessary to meet a person's need for energy*
> * *Variety in diet: Nutritious from diverse sources*

Growth

It is the gradual increase in size of the body, especially in terms of height and weight (9). It actually starts from conception, continues during the gestational period and then through infancy, childhood and adulthood;

however, the rates of growth among these periods differ substantially. In children, there is an overall quicker rate of growth, whereas in adults it is relatively very slow.

Development

It is the associated process in which there is an increase in the number and quality of skills performed by the body (4). Both of these concepts are part of one whole, forming a unified inseparable concept of growth and development. One of the reliable methods for measuring growth is Anthropometry.

FAILURE TO THRIVE
Any child who does not measure up to age appropriate growth and development standards is termed as his / her failure to thrive. Such children may be beset with, feeding difficulties, detached behaviour, sleep disturbances, difficulty in being comforted, hesitancy in social interactions and failure to gain weight etc. Several reasons can be attributed to this condition, for example:

- *Persistent ignorance of the child's basic physical needs (e.g. nutrition, housing and protection from assault)*
- *Persistent ignorance of the child's basic emotional needs (e.g. care, affection and stimulation)*
- *Neurological defects (e.g. mental retardation, tumour, infection etc.)*
- *Genetic disorders (e.g. chromosomal disorders, inborn errors of metabolism etc.)*
- *Miscellaneous causes (e.g. immunodeficiency disorders, intestinal obstruction etc.)*

These children may be able to thrive with appropriate diet and emotional support, and treatment of the underlying disease, if any.

Nutritional Needs

Nutritional needs during pregnancy

A pregnant woman needs extra energy and nutrition to meet the demands of her own body and the demand of the rapidly growing foetus which is entirely dependent on the mother's food. An estimate of the amount of growth and development during pregnancy could be made by just considering the change from one cell to millions of cells making a normal baby of about 3 Kg weight during the period of nine months. The mother's food habits and nutritional status during pregnancy greatly influence the health and growth of the baby. A healthy diet will provide all the essential nutrients and energy in sufficient quantities (10).

- Weight gain in pregnancy is closely related to the infant birth weight.
- Diet during pregnancy should include enough calories to meet high-energy demands and ensure adequate weight gain.
- Variety is the key to a healthy diet. It should include foods from each nutritional group.
- The rapid growth of baby during pregnancy needs a large amount of proteins. These could be provided with a combination of plant foods, if meat is unaffordable.
- Green leafy vegetables and fresh fruits should be eaten daily to provide sufficient minerals and vitamins.
- Use iodized salt to prevent mental disorders in baby.

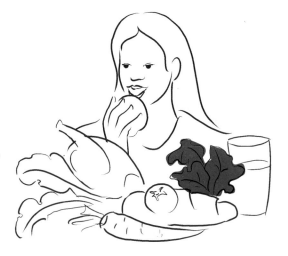

GROWTH:
Process characterized by increase in body size.

DEVELOPMENT:
Process involved in enhancing functional capabilities.

$\mathcal{T}$he brain grows, but the ability to reason develops.

DIETARY SUPPLEMENTS
Any commercial product intended to supplement the day-to-day diet.
Common Dietary Supplements are:
- *Multivitamins*
- *Minerals*
- *Fish oils and fatty acids*
- *Herbs and other plant extracts*

ANTENATAL CARE:
care provided to a woman during pregnancy by trained and skilled health personnel (doctors, nurses, midwives).

MATERNAL MALNUTRITION

In case of maternal nutritional deficiency there are increased risks of

- *Stillbirth*
- *Congenital abnormalities*
- *Pre-maturity*
- *Low birth weight*
- *Poor growth and development of foetus and*
- *Infant death during the first year of life*

- As iron is needed in large quantities and dietary supply cannot completely provide the needed amount, additional demands of iron could be met with iron supplements.
- The woman's body should be exposed daily to sunlight, which will provide vitamin D.
- Two glasses of milk should be taken daily to ensure adequate calcium and protein intake.
- 6-8 glasses of water should be taken daily to maintain adequate fluid volume, and to avoid constipation.

IRON DEFICIENCY

A disorder that results from a depletion of iron stores in the body. It can occur especially in women during pregnancy and due to inadequacy of weaning in infants. It is characterized by

- *Weakness*
- *Fatigue*
- *Short attention span*
- *Poor appetite*
- *Increased susceptibility to infection*
- *Irritability*

ECD REINFORCEMENTS

Special consideration for pregnancy

Avoid pregnancy in extreme ages

Pregnancy during older or very young age is an increased risk for the mother as well as the infant.

Provide social support during pregnancy

High levels of anxiety or stress in the mother may also increase the risk of complications of pregnancy or difficulties in the infant.

Place of delivery

Delivery at home under the supervision of a trained midwife is as safe as hospital delivery in case of uncomplicated, low risk pregnancies.

ECD REINFORCEMENTS

Nutrients and energy requirements are even greater during lactation than in pregnancy.

Nutritional needs during lactation

Considering the nutritive value of breast milk and its average daily production of 20-30 ounces each day the need for a balanced and adequate diet for a lactating woman cannot be over emphasized. Successful lactation is dependent upon increased diet, adequate fluids, rest, exercise and relaxation.

Tobacco or alcohol should not be used by a lactating woman. Use of medications needs to be avoided without the advice of a health care provider. Lactating women should try to get all of the nutrients they need from food, instead of from dietary supplements (10).

COLOSTRUM

Definition: Colostrum is the yellowish milk produced during the first few days (first three days 3 or so) after delivery.

Composition: proteins, minerals and antibodies are more than in the milk produced later.

Importance: high nutritive and disease protection qualities.

Nutritional needs during infancy (0 -2 years)

Food preferences of infants are moulded by the frequency and presentation of a particular food. Principally infants develop a rhythm in the need for feeding which falls into roughly 3-4 hour interval and this is known as self-demand feeding. This inter-feeding interval increases with age. Self demand feeding is preferable to the force feeding the child. A mother's skill in recognizing when her infant is hungry forms the basis for the success of self-demand feeding (8, 10).

a)   Weaning
Introducing solid foods

- **From birth to six months of age,** breast milk is sufficient to meet all the energy needs of an infant.

- **Six months** New foods should be introduced to the infant.
  Weaning should be initiated with a single food having easy digestibility e.g. rice cereal. Infants should be offered only one new food at a time. Any new food introduction should be made several days apart to pick up allergic reactions if any. Gradually introduce variety from each group of foods. Give small amounts of any new food at the beginning e.g., a teaspoonful or even less. Initially use foods of smooth consistency, gradually making it more solid. Gradually substitute finely chopped foods for strained foods (5, 8, 10).

- **Nine to twelve months** Mashed food should be started such as mashed potatoes, ripe banana, yogurt etc.

- **Twelve months onwards** Infants are ready to eat the same type of food as the rest of the family eats; yet these need to be mashed or cut up into small pieces and should be kept low in spices. Increase the variety of food. The desire for food progressively decreases in comparison to the first year; care givers should be reassured about the normality of this phenomenon and be educated to utilize food with high nutritive value for the child (5, 8, 10).

b)   Preparing weaning foods

- **Fruits:** Use clean, ripe fruits e.g. ripe bananas, pears, peaches, apricots. Wash thoroughly, peel off the fruit skin and mash with fork/spoon if the fruit is soft or mix in blender/pestle and mortar, if the food is hard
- **Vegetables:** Wash thoroughly; remove stem, seeds and skin. Boil or steam until soft. Mash and then offer to the infant.
- **Meats:** Cook meat (for example chicken, mutton, beef) thoroughly until soft. Remove fat, grind with water to make a puree and then offer to the infant.

If a refrigerator is available prepared weaning food could be frozen for a maximum of three days but the left over from the infant's dish should be discarded to avoid contamination(8).

c)   Consequences of Delayed Weaning
Weaning should be started at the age of six months. It is well established that late weaning is a major problem for the health of children, since breast-milk ceases to be adequate to meet the infants' needs between the ages of four and six months, and the risk of growth faltering and malnutrition is heightened from delayed weaning. In addition the infant's reserves of iron are usually depleted by the age of six months and they need additional source/s of iron. If weaning is delayed then infants are prone to develop micronutrient deficiencies especially iron deficiency anaemia, which in turn is manifested as irritability, fatigue, and poor appetite; in the long run these children have poor motor and mental development (8, 11).

Nutritional needs during early childhood (3-5 years)
During this period, the child develops better attention span and increased muscle coordination, but still

---

WEANING
means to discontinue breast-feeding and gradually substitute other feeding habits.
After six months, introduction of nutrient sources other than breast milk initiates weaning.

ECD REINFORCEMENTS
Prerequisites for weaning diet:

Person: Wash hands with soap and water

Place: Clean the surface where food is to be prepared

Utensils and equipment: Clean all the utensils (for example cup, spoon, plate, bowl, cooking pot) and equipment (for example blender, pestle and mortar).

finds some difficulties in handling food. This can be improved with proper encouragement during meal time.

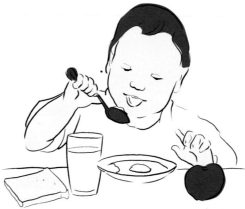

In order to fulfil the increased milk requirement, flavoured milk or milk-based foods can be offered such as kheer, custard, firni, pudding, and yogurt. Food given to the child should be lukewarm because children don't like extremes of temperature. Plain, bland and unmixed foods are preferred by the children of this age group.

The three meal schedule used by the rest of the family members, with the addition of midmorning and mid afternoon snacks forms an appropriate nutritional scheme for preschoolers (8, 10, 11).

Nutritional needs during middle childhood (6-10 years)

During these years of life, appetite is usually good. Breakfast should be given before sending the child to school. The amount of milk should be greater than that given to adults.

Children become willing to try those foods with friends which they do not like to eat alone. They are at particular risk of communicable diseases which cause dislike for food on the one hand, but have increased demand for food on the other. The child should be given foods which he/she likes to eat during the school break. Purchase of food from street vendors should not be allowed (8, 10, 11).

Food Preferences

Parents are often concerned regarding the diet of their children and their disinterest in eating. Forceful feeding is more likely to be unsuccessful and harmful for the child, and therefore it is important to understand the factors responsible for starting and stopping the need for food. A host of physiologic, environmental and social factors are responsible for intake of food, for example, presence of colourful, aromatic and appetizing food, other people who are eating and often the time for eating makes a child start eating.

The preference for the type and consistency of food is very much dependent on the age of the child. Children like a smooth consistency, with less spices and flavour in the food. Often watching other siblings and friends eating make them want to eat. In case of infants the caregiver's ability to recognize the baby's hunger is important, as infants usually establish a particular pattern for their feeding. In addition, the brain detects the signals of low status of energy and nutrients in diet and makes a person feel hunger and seek food. Satiety is the major factor stopping the child from eating, as nature indicates through the mechanisms of eyes, nose, throat, stomach and intestines that food is sufficient for the body for that point in time. Further dislike shown by parents or others for the child's food, too large a quantity, or a particular type of food served too often, also makes a child avoid that food.

These likes and dislikes develop because of cultural background and learning experiences. The food selection is also governed by sensory characteristics such as taste, smell, colour and temperature. The type of food offered, the way in which the food is presented and the frequency with which the food is offered contribute to food preferences. Over dosing with a particular food may provoke a dislike for that particular food for a long time. Also new foods should be gradually offered (8, 10, 12).

Why is my child not eating well?

It is usually a primary concern for a majority of caregivers. It is important for them to understand certain dietary principles for growing children.

- ### Children should decide how much to eat
  Children are born with regulatory processes that help them to decide how much to eat.

- ### Parents alone should decide as to which foods to offer to children
  Children are not born with any knowledge of the foods they should eat.

- ### Food preferences can and do change
  Food habits are learned from the assortment of food being offered to the child (13).

If a child dislikes a particular food, restrict that food item for some days and then try it again. Offering a food at different times in different combinations improves acceptance of the food.

ECD REINFORCEMENTS
Healthy food preferences to the child
1. *Offer only nutritious food choices.*
   There are no in-born mechanisms that enable children themselves select a nutritious diet.
2. *Offer variety of age appropriate nutritious food choices.*
   Infants learn to eat a variety of healthy foods by being offered a range of diets.
3. *Infants must be allowed to eat when they are hungry and to stop eating when they are full.*
4. *Offer food in a pleasant environment.*
5. *Give positive personal attention at the time of dining.*
6. *Food should not be used as a reward, penalty, or pacifier.*
7. *Infants or children should never be pressurized into eating anything.*
8. *Offer nutritious home based snacks in between meal times.*
9. *Food preferences change throughout childhood.*

ECD REINFORCEMENTS
Desired Healthy Diet Practices for Community Level Initiatives
Increase rates of:
- *Healthy weight gain in pregnancy*
- *Dietary supplements during pregnancy*
- *Age appropriate adequate breastfeeding*
- *Age appropriate adequate weaning*
- *Iodized salt*
Reduce dietary intake of:
- *Saturated fat e.g. banaspati ghee, clarified butter*
Increase dietary intake of:
- *Milk and dairy products*

ECD REINFORCEMENTS
Desired Healthy Diet Strategies for Community Level Initiatives
- *Provide nutrition counselling*
- *Enlarge growth monitoring activities*
- *Increase nutrition education in schools*
- *Enhance food security*
- *• Improve food safety and hygiene practices*

As a rule, children dislike foods which are said to be good for them, or are forced on them, and they take strong fancies to foods which they are not allowed to eat; advantage should be taken of these tendencies.
-Eric Pritchard

As a child my family's menu consisted of two choices: take it or leave it.
-Buddy Hackett

- *Fruits and vegetables*
- *Grain (e.g. wheat, rice, lentils)*

Food Allergy

Food allergies are more common in infants and young children in comparison to adults, because of their immature gastrointestinal tract. The symptoms of food allergy may vary from common diarrhoea, rash, congestion, runny nose to severe anaphylactic shock The importance of prevention and identification of food allergies lies in the fact that if a basic food component is known to cause allergy, appropriate dietary consult should be taken to substitute the body's demand with an alternative source and to prevent deficiency of that specific nutrient.

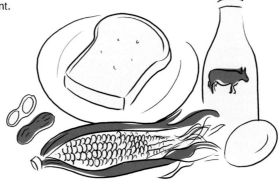

In order to prevent allergic reactions it is recommended that allergy creating foods should be eliminated from the infant's diet during the first year of life. By the time the child is 2-3 years old they usually outgrow their allergy and then these foods can gradually be given, but look for any allergic reaction (8, 11).

Food Taboos

While giving nutrition counselling to the caregiver, cultural values should especially be given consideration. Knowledge of locally available and acceptable food is very important for anyone concerned with nutrition counselling.

> *An onion can make people cry, but there has never been a vegetable invented to make them laugh.*
> -Will Rogers

Foods contrary to cultural values and beliefs are strongly rejected. No matter how balanced and adequate the diet plan is, it is not going to work if it is not acceptable in a particular culture. For example, use of shrimps, lobsters and other seafood for provision of proteins may strongly be rejected in certain communities.

The concept of 'hot' and 'cold' food refers to intrinsic quality rather than temperature. Examples of food considered 'hot' include eggs, fish, mango, while cold food include rice, banana and yogurt etc. 'Hot' foods are usually avoided if the child is suffering from diarrhoea. Similarly rice, banana and yogurt are avoided in respiratory problems, owing to their perception of 'cold' foods. It is important not to reject caregiver's beliefs regarding various foods outright. There are several ways to play around the perception of nutritionally valuable foods. For example, mango is considered 'hot' but is thought to become 'cold' if soaked in water for some time. Yogurt could be replaced with other milk products.

> *Vegetables are interesting but lack a sense of purpose when unaccompanied by a good cut of meat.*
> -Fran Lebowitz

It is a common practice to restrict the diet of children during illness. This should not be done, because that is the time when a child needs more nutrients: as a general rule two extra meals besides the recommended food for that particular age group should be given.

It is also widely believed that very little food should be given to pregnant woman to ensure the birth of a small baby, which is easy to deliver. In addition, neglect of the nutrition of a girl child is very common in rural and uneducated communities. It is important to recognize that the nutrition of a girl child is important than the nutrition of a baby boy, as she will be a mother and if malnourished will produce to a malnourished child and perpetuating, thus the vicious cycle of malnutrition that will run through generations(12).

Alternative sources of nutrition

No single food is a must for a child, except breastfeeding. Energy and nutrient demands of rapidly growing and developing children could be met through a number of cost effective alternatives.

- Meat, eggs and milk are considered expensive protein sources and their inclusion in the diet depends largely on affordability. Equivalent and cost effective nutritive benefits can be achieved through combination of certain plant foods e.g.
  - Rice and black beans
  - Rice and green peas
  - Bread (wheat) and green peas
  - Bread (wheat) and lentils
  - Various lentils cooked together
  - Corn and black eyed peas
- Similarly carrots, dates, guavas can easily be substituted for apples.
- Home gardening should be adopted to ensure easy availability of various vegetables and fruits at a small cost.

Anthropometry

The term **anthropometry** is made up of two words, i.e. *'Anthrop'* means **'man'** and *'metry'* means **'measurement'**. Hence, anthropometry is the measurement of the physical dimensions and gross composition of the body including its size, weight, and proportions of different parts (14).

Recognition of the effect of nutrition on human growth and development has made accurate measurement of the body indispensable for nutritional assessment, and the most commonly used, inexpensive and non-invasive method for this purpose is anthropometry. In childhood, under-nutrition is the single most important cause of growth retardation. Severe under-nutrition during the early phases of growth may considerably reduce the size of organs and thus the size of the body. The results of anthropometric measurements are then compared with values of a large number of healthy children of the same gender and age (4).

Anthropometric Measurements

Anthropometric measurements are sensitive indicators of health, nutrition and growth status of infants and children. The interpretation of anthropometric measurements is done through anthropometric indices that are made by combining two measurements, for example height and weight, to give a meaningful result.

In children, the three most commonly used anthropometric indices are (14):

i. **Weight-for-height:** reflects body weight relative to height. If the child is gaining insufficient weight relative to height, or is losing weight, he or she comes under the label of low weight for height or *Wasting*.

ii. **Height-for-age:** reflects whether the height is appropriate for age or not. If the child is gaining insufficient height relative to age it is referred to as *Stunting*.

iii. **Weight-for-age:** reflects body mass relative to age. If the child is gaining insufficient weight relative to age, or is losing weight, that child is considered *Underweight*.

The beet is the most intense of vegetables. The radish, admittedly, is more feverish, but the fire of the radish is a cold fire, the fire of discontent, not of passion. Tomatoes are lusty enough, yet there runs through tomatoes an undercurrent of frivolity. Beets are deadly serious.
    -Tom Robbins

BASIC COMPONENTS OF ANTHROPOMETRIC ASSESSMENT
- *Measuring the child*
- *Recording of the measurement*

Anthropometric assessments help in referral of infants/children with extremely low or high weight, length /height, or head circumference measurements

ANTHROPOMETRIC ASSESSMENTS REQUIRE
- *accurate equipments*
- *consistent techniques*
- *trained assessors*

Wasting indicates recent or continuing current severe weight loss.

Stunting is a consequence of long term sub-optimal health and nutrition.

Underweight is a composite indicator reflecting both recent and long-term malnutrition but can not distinguish between the two.

These simple measurements help in selecting individuals, families and communities for interventions designed to improve not only nutrition but health in general also.

Deficits of any of the above-mentioned indices are regarded as evidence of poor nutrition. With the help of these anthropometric indicators, past, present and future nutritional status can be assessed. Undernourished children do not grow to their full potential of mental and physical abilities, as is reflected by measurements below of standard cut off requirements. Information on underweight (low weight for age), stunting (low height for age) and wasting (low weight for height) are obtained from measurements of height and weight, by correlating these with age or with each other (10).

Protocol for anthropometric measurements in children

General Guidelines

- Examination should not interfere with the child's sleep, diet, or defecating activities. If the child is unwell at the time of visit, assess some time later.
- The child should be calm (not crying or irritable) at the time of examination.
- Record the measurements in pencil, and in case an error is made, completely erase the error and rewrite the correct numbers.
- Keep the pencil out of your mouth or hair when you weigh and measure, so that neither the child nor you can get hurt.
- Take measurements after verbal information has been noted down.
- Unbraid any hair that would interfere with the height measurement. Similarly, objects such as pins should be removed from the hair while taking head circumference.
- Hold the child firmly but gently.
- Make a consistent pattern of assessments under standardized conditions.
- Don't ever leave a child unattended.
- Take measurements with clean hands and clean scales.
- Take measurements in a room with sufficient light and comfortable temperature.

Prerequisite Information

Before moving to actual taking of measurements, the determination of the age and sex of the child is important.

- The first and most reliable way of finding out the age of the child is to look up the records from the health facilities (birth certificate, delivery card, etc). Verbal information from the primary caregiver should be considered as a second choice.
- If no such record exists, the data collector should first determine the year of birth by asking the mother if her child was born a few months before or after the birth of another child in the neighbourhood whose date of birth is known.
- To determine the month of birth, a local events calendar should be used.

Prerequisite Resources

a) Material Required

- Infant Weighing Scale
- Bathroom Scale
- Stadiometer (length measuring board)
- Measuring Tape (flexible and non-stretchable)
- Arm circumference insertion tape
- Growth Chart
- Pencil and Eraser

b)   Human Resources Required

- **Assessor:** responsible for taking the measurements.
- **Assistant:** responsible for assisting the assessor and will record the measurements on the growth chart.

If the assistant is untrained e.g. a primary caregiver, then the assessor should take the weight, head and mid upper arm circumference, and should record the measurements on the chart.

Parameters of Growth

i.   Weight
ii.   Height
iii.   Head circumference
iv.   Mid -upper arm circumference

Weight

Body weight is one of the most important measurements in nutritional assessment. It is also a valuable indicative measure of a child's growth. The parameter of growth reflects inadequate nutrition quickly. Response to an intervention could also be assessed through it. Weight increases rapidly during the first five years of life.

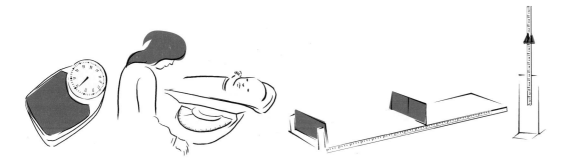

WEIGHING SCALE
- *There are many scales used for weighing, e.g. spring scale (Salter), beam balance and bathroom scales, etc.*
- *We prefer the infant weighing scale and bathroom (stand-on) scale because these are accurate, light, fairly reliable and portable.*
- *Infant weighing scale has an attached large tray for placement of the infant.*
- *It has a dial, which shows weight in kilograms, as well as in pounds.*
- *There are two needles; the longer needle shows weight from 0-10 kgs and the shorter one hows from 11-20 kg. If the child's weight is more than 10 kgs then the longer needle reaches the end point of 10 kg mark and disappears, while the shorter needle shows the weight.*
- *If the child is unable to stand, use an infant weighing scale and if the child is able to stand then use a bathroom scale.*

LOW BIRTH WEIGHT

Definition: Infants born weighing less than 2500 grams (2.5 kg)

Primary reason: Maternal malnutrition

Primary consequences:
- *Poor physical growth*
- *Delayed mental development*
- *Learning disabilities*
- *Death*

Advice:
- *Close contact with the caregiver*
- *Colostrum*
- *Regularly breast feed, if required, use expressed milk and feed with the help of cup and spoon*

HOW TO MEASURE WEIGHT ACCURATELY

1. Place the weighing scale against a smooth surface (table/ground). Make sure that the scale is stable and balanced.
2. Remove child's clothing and shoes (infants should be weighed nude or only with a diaper but older children could be weighed wearing light clothing)
3. Assessor: Adjust the pointer to zero before placing the infant/child on the scale
4. Assessor: Position the infant or child on the centre of the scale (make sure that the child does not touch any person or surrounding objects while being weighed).
5. Assessor: Check the infant/child's position and when correct, read and call out the measurement to the nearest 0.01 kg.
6. Assistant: Immediately record the measurement and show it to the assessor.
7. Assessor: Check the recorded measurement on the paper for accuracy and legibility. Instruct the assistant to erase and correct any errors.

Table 1: Expected normal values for weight at various ages (11, 12)

Age	Expected Normal Weight*
Birth	3 kg
6 months	8 kg
1 year	10 kg
2 years	12 kg
3 years	14 kg
4 years	16 kg
5 years	18 kg
6 years	20 Kg

* Rounded off for simplicity

Length/Height

Measurement of height is one of the most fundamental and easily obtained anthropometric measurements. In addition to weight, the child's height is another useful indicator of growth. Length refers to the measurement in recumbent (lying down) position and height to measurement in standing position. Serial length /height measurements can be used to detect growth retardation if they are made at long intervals (3 to 6 months).

STADIOMETER
- *For measurement of height, a specific instrument called a Stadiometer is used.*
- *It comprises of a vertical board, with a movable horizontal headpiece*
- *A metric rule is attached to the vertical board*

LENGTH MEASURING BOARD
- *For measuring the length of infants, a specific scale, a length measuring board, is used.*
- *It has a firm, flat horizontal surface with a fixed head piece and a movable foot piece.*
- *Measurement tape/ markings are present longitudinally on one side of the board.*

CAUTION
Length/height should not be measured from the weighing scales having attached device for length/height.

How to measure height accurately (15, 16)

1. Place the measuring board against a smooth surface. Make sure that the board is stable.
2. Ask the mother to remove the child's shoes and ask her to walk the child to the board and to kneel

LENGTH
- *Height measurement technique for infants is known as "Length"*
- *Length is taken in recumbent position.*

STATURE
- *Height measurement technique for children is known as "Stature",*
- *Stature is taken in standing position.*

n front of the child.

3. Assistant: Place the paper and pencil on the ground, and kneel with both knees on the right side of the child.

4. Assessor: Kneel on your right knee, on the child's left side.

5. Assistant: Place the child's feet flat and together in the centre of and against the back and base of the board. Place your right hand just above the child's ankles on the shins; place your left hand on the child's knees and push against the board. Make sure the child's legs are straight and the heels and calves are against the board. Tell the assessor when you have completed positioning the feet and legs.

6. Assessor: Tell the child to look straight ahead at the mother, if she is in front of the child. Make sure the child's line of sight is level with the ground. Place your open left hand on the child's chin. Gradually close your hand. Make sure the shoulders are level, the hands are at the child's side, and head, shoulder blades and buttocks are against the board. With your right hand, lower the headpiece on the top of the child's head. Make sure you push through the child's hair.

7. Assessor and Assistant: Check the child's position. Repeat any necessary steps.

8. Assessor: When the child's position is correct, read and call out the measurement to the nearest 0.1 cm. Remove the headpiece from the child's head, your left hand from the child's chin and support the child during the recording.

9. Assistant: Immediately record the measurement and show it to the assessor.

10. Assessor: Check the recorded measurement on the paper for accuracy and legibility. Instruct the assistant to erase and correct any errors.

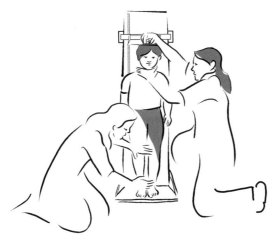

How to Measure Length Accurately (15, 16)

1. Place the measuring board on a hard flat surface i.e. ground, floor or steady table.

2. Assistant: Place the paper and pencil on the ground, floor or table. Kneel with both knees behind the base of the board, if it is on the ground.

3. Assessor: Kneel on the right side of the child, so that you can hold the foot piece with your right hand

4. Assistant: with the primary caregiver's help, lay the child on the board, then support the back of the child's head with your hands, and gradually lower the child on to the board.

5. Assessor: Ask the primary caregiver to kneel on the opposite side of the board facing the measurer to help keep the child calm.

6. Assistant: Cup your hands over the child's ears. With your arms comfortably straight, place the child's head against the base of the board so that the child is looking straight up. The child's line of sight should be perpendicular to the ground. Your head should be straight over the child's head. Look

QUALITY ASSURANCE IN ANTHROPOMETRIC ASSESSMENT
- *Weighing scales: checked, zeroed (scale showing zero reading without any weight) and tested with standard weights every time the scales are moved.*
- *Length boards and Stadiometer: checked and tested with standard length rods every time these are moved.*
- *Assessor: trained by someone trained and experienced in performing anthropometric assessments.*

directly into the child's eyes.

7. Assessor: Make sure the child is lying flat and in the centre of the board. Place your left hand on the child's shins (above the ankles) or on the knees. Press them firmly against the board. With your right hand, place the foot piece firmly against the child's heels.

8. Assessor: Check the child's position. Repeat any necessary steps.

9. Assessor: When the child's position is correct, read and call out the measurement to the nearest 0.1 cm. Remove the foot piece, release your left hand from shin or knees of the child and support him/her during the recording.

10. Assistant: Immediately release the child's head, record the measurement, and show it to the assessor.

11. Assessor: Check the recorded measurement on the paper for accuracy and legibility. Instruct the assistant to erase and correct any errors.

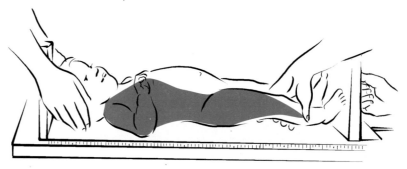

PRECISION OF ANTHROPOMETRIC MEASUREMENTS

- *Weight = 0.01 kg*
- *Length/stature = 0.1 cm*
- *Head Circumference = 0.1 cm*

Table 2: Expected normal values for length/height at various ages (11, 12)

Age	Parameter	Expected average values*
Birth	Length	50 cms
6 months	Length	68 cms
1 year	Length	76 cms
2 years	Length	87 cms
3 years	Height	96 cms
4 years	Height	103 cms
5 years	Height	110 cms
6 years	Height	116 cms
after the age of 2 years until puberty the average gain in height is 5-7.5 cms per year		

* Rounded off for simplicity

Head Circumference

Measurement of head circumference (Occipitofrontal Circumference-OFC) is an important screening procedure to detect abnormalities of head and brain growth, particularly in the first year of life, which may or may not be related to nutritional factors.

Head circumference increases rapidly during the first twelve months of life but by thirty six months growth is much slower. It is often used in clinical settings as part of health screening for potential development or for detecting neurological disabilities in children.

When to measure Head Circumference

Ideally, the first measurement should be recorded two to four days after birth as a base line for future measurements. It should be measured routinely on infants/children up to age 36 months.

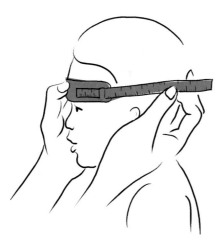

HEAD CIRCUMFERENCE MEASURING TAPE
- *Head circumference is measured with a flexible non-stretchable measuring tape*
- *The tape should be · -1/2 inch wide*
- *The tape should have 0.1 cm increments*

HOW TO MEASURE HEAD CIRCUMFERENCE ACCURATELY (15, 16)

1. *Assessor: Ask the primary caregiver of the child to hold the child in her lap. If the child is able to stand then the measurement could be taken in the standing position. The lower edge of the tape should be positioned just above the eyebrows, above (not over) the ears, and around the back of the head.*
2. *The tape should be in the same plane on both sides of the head and pulled slightly to compress the hair.*
3. *When the child's position is correct, read and call out the measurement to the nearest 0.1 cm. Remove the measuring tape from the child's head.*
4. *Assistant: Immediately record the measurement, and show it to the assessor.*
5. *Assessor: Check the recorded measurement on the paper for accuracy and legibility. Instruct the assistant to erase and correct any errors.*

Table 3: Expected Normal Values for OFC at various ages (11, 12)

Age	Expected Normal Value of OFC*
Birth	35 cms
3 months	40 cms
1 year	47 cms
2 years	49cms
3 years	50cms
6 years	59 cms

* Rounded off for simplicity

Mid-Upper Arm Circumference (MUAC)

This is another measurement used to assess nutritional status of children from 1-5 years of age as it stays at 16cm on average during this period. When children are about 1 year old they have quite a lot of fat under the skin of their arms. When they are 5 years old there is much less fat and more muscle. But the distance around the upper arm remains almost the same between the ages of 1 and 5 years (11). If the child is malnourished, this circumference is reduced. A single cut-off value, usually 12.5 cm, is taken and any measurement below this indicates malnutrition.

In malnutrition, MUAC decreases (12).
- *Above 1 year, if MUAC is between 13.5-16 cm = normal.*
- *Above 1 year, if MUAC is between 12.5-13.5 cm = borderline malnutrition.*
- *Above 1 year, if MUAC is below 12.5 cm = severe malnutrition.*

When to measure MUAC

If the age of the child is between 1 and 5 years, and in conditions where measurements of height and weight are difficult to obtain for example, in emergencies like refugee crises and drought, etc.

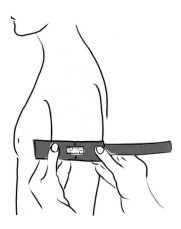

HOW TO MEASURE MUAC ACCURATELY (15)

The measuring tape should be used for measuring MUAC.

1. *Assessor: Ask the primary care giver to remove clothing that may cover the child's left arm. Calculate the mid point of the child's left upper arm by first locating the tip of the child's shoulder with your fingertips. Bend the child's elbow to make a right angle. Place the tape at the zero, which is indicated by two arrows on the tip of the shoulder and pull the tape straight down past the tip of the elbow. Read the number at the tip of the elbow to the nearest centimetre. Divide this number by two to estimate the midpoint. As an alternative, bend the tape up to the middle length to estimate the midpoint. Mark the midpoint with a pen on the arm. Straighten the child's arm and wrap the tape around the arm at the midpoint. Make sure the tape is flat around the skin. Inspect that tension of the tape on the child's arm is proper and is not too tight or too loose. Repeat any necessary steps.*
2. *Assistant: Have the paper and pencil ready.*
3. *Assessor: When the tape is in the correct position on the arm with the correct tension, read and call out the measurement to the nearest 0.1 cm.*
4. *Assistant: Immediately record the measurement on the paper and show it to the assessor.*
5. *Assessor: Check the recorded measurement on the paper for accuracy and legibility. Instruct the assistant to erase and correct any errors.*

Table 4: The expected normal values for MUAC at various ages (11, 12)

Age	MUAC
Birth	11 cms
1 year	16 cms
5 years	17 cms

Growth Monitoring and Promotion

Growth monitoring and promotion is a continuous activity with the goal of improving the health of children. The 'monitoring' part deals with the regular measurement and recording of a child's growth change and the 'promotion' part is related to the counselling of the caregiver regarding the health and nutrition of his/her child. It enables the caregivers to understand the growth pattern of their children and to take any actions, if required.

Growth monitoring and promotion is used to identify children who need supplementary food and treatment for disease. It is also used to monitor the growth of children who are diagnosed with malnutrition. In order to check the responses of malnourished children after intervention, growth monitoring is used. The unique feature of growth monitoring and promotion is that it involves caregivers in monitoring the growth of their children (17).

Growth Charts and Nutritional Counselling

The growth chart is one of the tools for growth monitoring and promotion. The World Health Organization has recommended the growth charts developed by the Centres for Disease Control to be used internationally (18). (see Appendix III). . Race and ethnicity specific growth charts are not developed as growth is the fundamental human characteristic and variations are largely attributed to environmental factors. The real benefit from plotting growth charts depends upon accurate, periodic measurements of children. These charts indicate at a glance whether the child is growing well or not. The reference lines show percentiles (uppermost line shows 95th percentile, middle shows 50th percentile and lower most line shows 5th percentile). If for example a child's weight for age comes on 50th percentile, it means that weight of the 50 percent children of the similar age fall below their values. If any child's weight measurements fall in the topmost percentile, line percentile (i.e. 95th) it means the child's weight is greater than or equal to the measurements of 95% of children of that age. The remaining 5% of children of that age have weight measurements that exceed that child's. Such a child is known as having obesity. The caregivers need to be informed about the dietary modification that the child will require, rather than depriving the child of meals. In that regard food rich in calories, fried and junk food need to be avoided, and greater emphasis placed on fruit and vegetables in addition to milk and other protein containing food which are necessary for rapidly growing children.

As children grow, their needs for energy and nutrients change. They need large amounts of energy, protein, vitamins, and minerals to support their tremendous growth and development. Since the feeding of children is largely dependent on their primary caregivers, education should be designed to guide them to provide a balanced diet to the growing child. For the growth promotion of a child, it is essential that the findings of growth monitoring should be shared with primary caregivers. They should be counselled that an extremely high or low reading means there is a problem. For example if a child's weight falls in the 5th percentile, that means 95% of children of that age weigh more and 5% weigh less than that child. Such a child will be malnourished; the caregivers are counselled to increase the diet of the child. For counselling skills, see relevant section in the chapter of communication skills. It is also important to refer the children with extremely high or low anthropometric assessment values for further evaluation by a health care provider.

Generally, if a measurement exceeds the 50th and is closer to the 95th percentile line than the 50th percentile line, there is chance for that child to be overweight. On the other hand, if a measurement falls below the 50th percentile line or is closer to the 5th percentile line than the 50th percentile line, then the child is likely to be underweight.

It is very important not to focus on a single reading of growth charts. For example, a child's height measurement might place him near the 5th percentile, but this usually doesn't indicate a growth problem if his/her subsequent measurements continue to track along the same percentile (as might be possible if a child's parents are also short in height). If the community worker and parents consider a single measurement, they might wrongly worry about the child's growth. When growth chart readings are examined over time, they reveal a pattern of development. That pattern reveals the growth of a particular child in relation to other children of his age. Serial measurements also shows how a child has progressed from previous measurements (14, 18).

GROWTH MONITORING
It is the process of regular anthropometric measurement, recording and interpretation of a child's growth change.

GROWTH PROMOTION
It is the regular process of using growth monitoring in order to counsel caregivers and enable them to increase control over and improve the growth of their children.

The 95th percentile is the upper and 5th percentile is the lower limit of normal growth

Anthropometric Assessments in the Context of Early Child Development

At Program Level

The notion of Early Child Development (ECD) has gained momentum during the past three decades. The early years of life are of heightened importance for the future productivity, health and intellectual potential of the child, because foundations for all these are laid during the initial period of life. The key concept of early child development programs is that an investment in children is an investment in the future. These programs are comprehensive and they deal with the several needs of a child whether physical, intellectual or mental (19).

The idea behind growth monitoring by anthropometry is to identify those children who are not growing normally and to classify their nutritional status so that appropriate intervention can be carried out. Field workers given sufficient training can assess growth by anthropometry. It is also important for field workers to have an understanding of theory behind anthropometric measurement techniques; they should also be proficient in their use of the various techniques. Assessment of nutritional status by anthropometry is one of the important indicators in ECD programs throughout the world. These programs not only emphasize the promotion of proper nutrition for growth and development but also recognize and deliver cost effective nutritional interventions.

Anthropometric assessment has several implications at the program level, for example:
- Defining the nutritional status for purposes of program planning, implementation and evaluation
- Selection of populations for participation in an intervention
- Prediction of benefits to be obtained from an intervention
- Evaluation of effects of changing nutritional, health or socioeconomic influences including interventions
- Identification of social or economic inequity, food insecurity, poverty.
- Depiction of community response to interventional program
- Provision of feedback to the management of the intervention programs
- Guidance for public health decision making
- Assessment of living standards of a community
- Comparison of the growth of children with different national and international populations of the same age and sex.

At Individual Level

Besides the numerous advantages of anthropometric assessments at the early child development program level, several implications exist for the individual child level.
- Anthropometry allows development with a view to nutrition and health status of an individual child
- Growth monitoring of a child could be done with the help of anthropometry
- Anthropometry highlights the need for referral of an individual; if his/her growth is not proceeding as expected.
- Anthropometric measurements form the basis of many clinical decisions by health care providers for an individual

Summary
- **Nutrition** is the science of composition of nutrients and their effects on health. There are six categories

of chemical substances found in food, which are called nutrients; these include carbohydrates, proteins, fats, vitamins, minerals and water.

- **A healthy diet** is characterized by balance, adequacy and variety. A diet which is either unbalanced or inadequate can result in malnutrition.

- **Two related concepts** with nutrition are growth and development. Growth is a process characterized by increase in body size and development by increase in functional capabilities.

- **Nutritional needs** vary during different phases of life. Both during pregnancy and lactation extra amount of energy and nutrients are needed to meet the increased demand. Maternal malnutrition during pregnancy is associated with adverse pregnancy outcomes.

- **During infancy** the first 6 months should include exclusive breastfeeding; thereafter, gradual introduction of semisolid food is recommended.

- **Food allergies** are common during infancy, usually resulting from cow's milk, eggs, wheat and nuts, therefore these foods should be introduced after the first year of life.

- **For the period of early childhood** (3-5 years), the three meal pattern followed by adults with the addition of mid morning and mid afternoon snacks fulfils the nutritional demands of preschoolers.

- **Age group (6-10 years)** comprises of school going children and breakfast and food during the school break should not be missed and greater requirements for milk should be met.

- **Intake of food** is very much dependent upon the food preferences which develop largely owing to the cultural background and learning experiences. Nutritional counselling should take care of cultural values and proper tackling of food fads and taboos.

- **Anthropometry** is the measurement of physical dimensions and gross composition of the body. It forms one of the important ways to assess the health and nutritional status of children. It serves as an important tool in the context of early child development both at the program and individual child level.

- **Most commonly used anthropometric parameters** for children include weight, height and head circumference. A combination of two anthropometric parameters forms the anthropometric indices which convert these measurements for meaningful information for several purposes. The term *Wasting* is used to describe weight loss of recent origin, *Stunting* results from malnutrition of long-term origin and *Underweight* is the composite index, which reflects both recent and long-term malnutrition but can not distinguish between the two.

- **Anthropometric assessments** require trained measurers, standardized techniques and accurate equipments.

- **The measurements taken** are plotted on a growth chart to compare with a reference population. A series of measurements over a period of time are reliable indicators of growth rather than a single measurement.

- **Counselling of caregivers** regarding basic principles of nutrition is very important from a child's health and growth perspective. Emphasis should be placed upon intake of a balanced and adequate

Bread is the king of the table and all else is merely the court that surrounds the king. The countries are the soup, the meat, the vegetables, the salad but bread is king.
-Louis Bromfield

The wise man should consider that health is the greatest of human blessings. Let food be your medicine.
Hippocrates

*The best six doctors anywhere
And no one can deny it
Are sunshine, water, rest, and air
Exercise and diet.
These six will gladly you attend
If only you are willing
Your mind they'll ease
Your will they'll mend
And charge you not a shilling.*
-Nursery rhyme quoted by Wayne Fields

*i*NTELLECTUAL

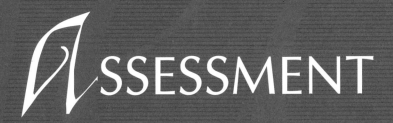

ASSESSMENT

A 3-year-old child Amir, is busy playing with different geometric shapes, which he has to fit in a pattern box. First, he tries to fit a circle in a square shaped hole, but he realizes that this is wrong; he then tries fitting it into a triangle shaped hole, and then after failing once again he finally fits it in the circle shaped hole. He laughs and is happy with his achievement. He continues filling all the shapes successfully in their respective holes.

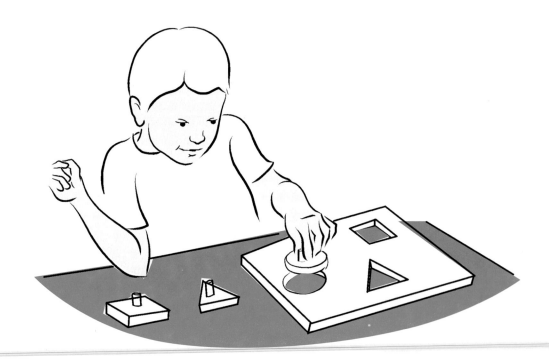

COMPETENCE:
Status of behaviour and skill demonstrated by a child under ideal conditions.

PERFORMANCE:
Status of behaviour and skill demonstrated by a child under real life conditions.

Direct measurement of competence is usually not possible; we typically measure performance in standardized real life conditions.

Now can we infer that this child is intelligent? First, it is better to understand what intelligence is.

Intelligence

Intelligence comes from the word intellect, which means the capacity of understanding, thinking and reasoning. Therefore, intelligence can be defined as the combination of inherited ability and environmental experiences, which result in a person's ability to acquire, retain and understand different concepts, to understand the relationship between objects, events, and ideas, and as the ability to apply this understanding in solving the problems of everyday life (1).

General Domains of Intelligence

These domains are interrelated. Nevertheless, classification enables appraisal of factors that may be especially important for the development assessed under each domain.

a)   Memory

It is the capacity of the mind to understand, store and retrieve information. Through this process, the child can also recognize the faces of people and objects (2).

If a mother shows a family photograph to her son and asks him, "Neha,I where is your sister in this photo?" he immediately points towards the face of his sister in the photo

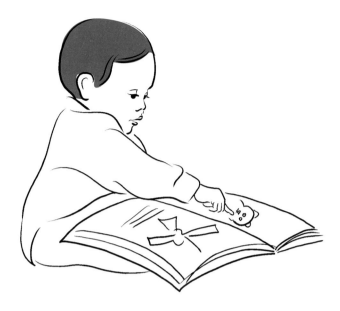

b)　Language

Language is the medium of communication through which one receives and conveys messages and communicates needs, feelings and opinions. It reflects learning and enables learning through communication (3). A language mainly comprises comprehension and production.

i.　Language Comprehension:

The language that the child understands

A 2-year-old boy, Yousaf, follows the simple directions of his mother, as she asks him to fetch his toy; Yousaf follows the request immediately.

ii.　Language Production:

It consists of the words and combination of words that children use.

"I need water" Yousaf communicates his need to his mother.

c)　Reasoning

It refers to a set of cognitive processes by which an individual may reach a conclusion from a collection of evidence, or from statements of principles. Thus, it is a process of drawing conclusions based on presented instances (4).

Sami, a 2 1/2-year-old child is playing with spoons and bowls; he sorts out similar objects by gathering the spoons in one place and the bowls in another.

d)　Problem Solving

It refers to a process of identifying and analyzing problems, discussing them and arriving at workable solutions, which can in turn be evaluated and improved in subsequent attempts. Primarily it is identifying

---

MEMORY

- *Say the nouns and keep asking similar questions from time to time.*
- •• *Ask the child to narrate past activities.*
- *Ask about daily life activities to keep track*

LANGUAGE

- *Talk in lengthy sentences*
- *Talk about everything present in the environment*
- *Tell stories to the child*
- *Emphasize various words used in the story*
- *Speak correctly and clearly.*
- *Listen carefully to the questions of the child and respond positively*
- *Ask the child to narrate any event*
- *Don't expect perfect grammar.*

"Too often we give our children answers to remember rather than problems to solve.
-Roger Lewin"

the means to achieve a result. Thus, it is a process through which an individual understands, defines and solves the problem.

Adam is playing with toys when his cousins come to visit. He knows that his cousins will also want to play with his toys, and may even break them, so he puts his toys away in a box, and hides this box under the bed.

e) Psychomotor

It is the capacity to relate muscular and mental activity. Psychomotor development refers to a child's control over his/her muscles, coordination, and ability to sit, stand, and eventually to walk and run. They affect sensory perception and learning through exploration and experience.

Reena is an 8 month old child, sitting in front of many colourful toys. She tries to grasp the rattle and using her psychomotor ability, transfers the rattle from one hand to the other.

i. **Fine Motor:** refers to small muscle movement and control i.e. use of small muscle groups for specific tasks such as stacking small blocks, stringing beads, tracking an object with the eyes, smiling and handwriting.

ii. **Gross motor:** refers to large muscle movement and control i.e. use of large muscle groups for specific tasks such as holding your head up, walking, running, skipping, climbing, jumping.

ECD REINFORCEMENTS

These milestones provide a guide to parents, telling them what to expect and when to expect it. Remember that departures from the norm should not be a reason for undue panic unless confirmed by expert medical opinion.

PSYCHOMOTOR
- *Opportunity to move freely under caregiver's supervision.*
- *Involve child in physical activities like sport.*
- ● ● *Encourage child to feed himself, draw and colour sketches etc.*

PHYSICAL DEVELOPMENT
- *New behaviours are triggered by changes in physical growth and development.*
- *Physical skills affect the kinds of experiences the child can have, and experience affects the child's feelings about her/his own body, self-concept and personality.*

f) Curiosity

It refers to a state in which you want to learn more about something. Exploratory behaviour is referred to as Curiosity, that is, the degree to which a child reacts to a new, strange and incongruous element in the environment. This could either be by observing the object, approaching the object, manipulating the object and finally asking questions about the object.

Gul is a 2-year-old child, observing his 5 year old elder sister Mona who is playing with a doll which produces sounds when moved. Soon his mother calls Mona. She leaves the doll on the floor and goes to her mother. In the meantime, Gul moves towards the doll and tries to move the doll to produce sounds just as his sister was doing. He starts looking for the cause of the sound while banging it, so

---

Infants develop gross motor control before they develop fine motor control

Psychomotor development proceeds from head to toe. Hence, the child first learns to control his head, then his body, arms and legs.

MOTOR DEVELOPMENT
- *Growth and change in capability to execute*
- *Gross motor skills such as crawling, walking or running*
- *Fine motor skills such as scribbling, drawing or writing*

CURIOSITY
- ● ● *Provide stimulating and supporting environment to explore through all of the senses.*
- ● ● *Avoid restricting the child from exploration; rather give support to search the environment under supervision.*
- ● ● *Respond positively to all your child's questions*

that he can get it to produce a sound. Soon Mona comes back and he asks her, where does this sound come from? How does this doll speak?

g)   Emotional State

This refers to the state of a person's emotions, especially with regard to pleasure or dejection. During observation, the child's emotional state can be practically noted as happy or passive. 'Happy' is the state when the child smiles and takes an interest in surrounding activities during most of the time of observation for intellectual assessment, whereas a passive state is that in which the child ignores surrounding activities, is unhappy or not sociable, or is even aggressive or hostile.

Tania, a class teacher at the day care center is to carry out the assessment: 2 1/2 year old Aamir, is playing with another child when Tania asks if would he like to colour the circle on the paper. He smiles and nods, and starts colouring. On the other hand, Asad, a boy of the same age is sitting all alone in a corner of the room, not taking interest in the other children's activities as he has quarrelled with someone. As the teacher approaches him, he turns his face away; when she tries to talk to him he just pulls back her as if he does not want to talk to her.

Now the question arises in one's mind as to whether intelligence is a single or multifaceted factor. It has been realized that intelligence is a multifaceted factor, which includes abilities that operate independently as well as in combination.

It is a common misconception that a child is intelligent if she/he holds a good position in class, whether she/he gets that position by comprehending the concepts of a subject or just by rote learning. A child could be good in painting or drawing but not good in arithmetic. It does not mean he is not intelligent. There are certain specific intellectual abilities, which vary from individual to individual (5). In addition, expectations and nurturing of specific intellectual abilities vary from culture to culture (6).

In rural areas, parents expect and nurture their sons to be physically strong and skillful so that they can start work early in life, share their father's responsibilities, and provide financial support in adulthood. In urban areas, parent's expectations are rather different: they focus on early schooling because they want their children to have control over reflexes, better reasoning and memory, and language ability with the help of which children can perform better in school.

Nature versus Nurture

Now the question arises as to how a child can be intelligent. There are two major factors which determine the intelligence of an individual i.e. heredity and environment (7).

Heredity

Intelligence is partly attributed to genes. Children inherit genes from their parents.

Hereditary defects and deficiencies can be minimized by preventing cousin marriages, which transfer the same gene from one generation to another. This custom is quite prevalent in developing countries.

Genetic make up cannot be changed once the child is born, but environment can be modified: this factor is also significant in the development of children's intelligence.

> *"Well," said Pooh, "what I like best," and then he had to stop and think. Because although Eating Honey was a very good thing to do, there was a moment just before you began to eat it which was better than when you were, but he didn't know what it was called.*
> *-A.A. Milne*

> *A young child is, indeed, a true scientist, just one big question mark. What? Why? How? I never cease to marvel at the recurring miracle of growth, to be fascinated by the mystery and wonder of this brave enthusiasm.*
> *-Victoria Wagner*

Environment

The environment consists of many factors, such as

a)   Health and Nutrition

A child's good health is related to enhancement of intellectual ability, especially through proper development of intelligence and ability to explore the environment.

b)   Stimulating Environment

The child gets stimulated through all his/her senses including touch, sight, hearing, smell and taste, which facilitate intellectual development. The time devoted by parents to talking to their children, playing, reading and story telling, helps to operate the child's mental faculties.

Communication is effective in helping children develop language. Similarly, to play with them not only establishes affectionate bonding between child and caregiver, but also helps the child to learn different skills like reading. Story telling develops curiosity and reasoning ability in a child. These qualities encourage him to explore the surrounding world.

> *The race that does not value trained intelligence is doomed.*
> -Alfred Whitehead

Importance of being Intelligent

Intelligence helps a person to:

- Adjust effectively to his/her environment.
- Develop the ability to learn and profit from experience.
- Effectively solve the problems of his/her daily life.
- Acquire professional skills that help in economic productivity.
- Enhance social adaptability.

> *It is a miracle that curiosity survives formal education.*
> -Albert Einstein

Measures of Intelligence

The concept of intelligence is not as concrete as physical concepts like height, weight, age etc. Intelligence cannot be measured directly, but can be measured by indirect estimation by evaluating the intelligent acts of a child. Usually the following tests are used for the assessment of the child's intellectual level.

- Baley Scale of Infant Development (BSID)
- Wechsler Preschool and Primary Scale of Intelligence (WPPSI)
- Stanford-Binet Intelligence Scale

The average time spent in assessment is from 25 to 60 minutes, and the age category ranges between 1 month to 14 years.

Conceptual understanding of some challenges encountered during the learning process of a child

> *Man paints with his brains and not with his hands.*
> -Michelangelo

Learning styles and intelligence

We all know that each child is unique, in temperament, physical appearance etc. but usually overlook this fact when children differ in their ways of learning too. Learning is a process of sensory perception and processing of information. Every individual has his/her preferred perceptions. Some respond to verbal instruction, some need visual aids for greater understanding, and some involve their bodies actively in their learning. Their preferred medium of learning is irrespective of their intellectual status. However, if a conducive environment is provided according to the respective learning style, then the child's intellectual status can be enhanced significantly. Based on perceptual modalities there are three basic learning styles:

a) Auditory (hearing the information)
The child prefers auditory information, and retains content that has been verbally communicated.

b) Visual (seeing the information)
The child prefers visual depiction of the information; and learns through images, enjoys art and drawing, reads maps, charts and diagrams well.

c) Kinesthetic- tactile (touching, participation)
The child prefers knowledge processes through physical sensations, is very active, and not able to sit still for long periods of time; communicates with body language and gestures, and she / he prepares to show, rather than tell stories, and need to touch and feels the world.

Caregivers play a vital role in enhancing the learning ability of the child by providing the opportunity to use his/her preferred modality. Usually caregivers teach in learning styles in which they are themselves comfortable, which may be different from the child's preferred learning style. This can be frustrating for both caregiver and child. Provide support by using a child's preferred sensory modality, so that the learning process becomes interesting and enjoyable not only for the child but also for the caregiver.

Because a child has a preferred perception modality, it does not mean that he/she has only one learning style: other modalities, which can enhance the learning process, can also be used.

CLASSROOM
Within the classroom, the focus should be on providing a learning environment based on stimulation of all sensory modalities, as the class usually represents students with varied learning styles. In this way, teaching with the use of all learning modalities can cater to the needs of all the students.

HOME
The caregiver should identify and focus on the specific perceptual needs of the child to make the learning process more efficient/effective.

Learning Disability and intelligence
Learning disability is a disorder which affects a child's ability to either adequately interpret what they see and hear, or to link the processed information from different parts of the brain. These limitations are characterized by difficulties in learning specific skills at the same rate as most people of the same age (8). There is typically a significant difference between academic achievement and intellectual ability. Disability involves:

- Having overall normal intelligence or above but incomplete development in one or more of intellectual domains.

AUDITORY LEARNING
- *Read any story or topic to the child*
- *let it be retained by asking questions or re-reading it aloud*

VISUAL LEARNING
- *Give picture books*
- *Encourage the visualization of scenes at intervals, while narrating an event*
- *Allow the child to make some reminder marks, e.g. stars, during writing*

KINESTHETIC-TACTILE LEARNING
- *Hands-on activities and experiments, such as art projects*
- *Nature walks*
- *Opportunities for acting out stories*

LEARNING DISABILITY
Most cases are best taken care of by intensive individually tailored one-to-one instruction in reading and writing.

GIFTED
A child's unexpected or unexplained skill or performance in
- *Mathematics*
- *Music*

*S*imran's overall academic performance is good as she always secures a position in an exam among first 10 students in the class, but her marks in arithmetic are always barely at passing grade.

- Having difficulties in at least one academic area, usually several, such as listening, speaking, reading, written expression, mathematics, and reasoning.

It does not include children who have learning problems, which are primarily the result of visual, hearing, or motor disabilities; mental retardation; emotional disturbance; or environmental, cultural, or economic disadvantages.

LEARNING DISABILITY (LD)
a child's unexpected or unexplained problem (neurological dysfunction) in learning to
- *Read*
- *Spell*
- *Calculate*

Significance of Intellectual Assessment in Relation to ECD

1. This helps to assess the age appropriate intellectual functioning of a child.

*N*ajma's mother worriedly commented that her daughter cannot speak even at the age of two. How can she make sure that everything is all right with Najma?

2. Provide insight about the abilities and skills of the child.

A test result reveals that if a child, Ahmed, is good in language, a suggestion can be given to the caregiver to provide him a conducive environment by having conversations with him or encouraging him to tell stories to enhance his ability.

3. Certain intelligence tests also indicate the presence of learning difficulties and disabilities. Based on that, supportive measures can be suggested.

Summary

- **Intelligence** comes from the word intellect, which means the capacity of understanding, thinking and reasoning.

- **Competence** is a status of behaviour and skill demonstrated by a child under ideal conditions.

- **Performance** is a status of behaviour and skill demonstrated by a child under real life conditions.

- **General Domains** of intelligence include memory, language, reasoning, problem solving, psychomotor abilities, curiosity and emotional state. These domains are interrelated and performance of these is also dependent upon the emotional state of the child, especially with regard to pleasure or dejection.

- **Nature and Nurture** act interdependently in determining the intellectual development of the child. Each child is born with specific inborn qualities and abilities (nature), while they are pruned back and groomed according to individual variation in the environment, available to each child (nurture).

- **Learning** is a process of sensory perception and processing of information.

- **Learning style** of an individual is based on the preferred sensory perceptions for learning. There

*T*his I believe: that the free, exploring mind of the individual human is the most valuable thing in the world. And this I would fight for: the freedom of the mind to take any direction it wishes, undirected. And this I must fight against: any idea, religion, or government which limits or destroys the individual.
-John Steinbeck

are three basic types: Auditory (hearing the information), Visual (seeing the information) and Kinesthetic- tactile (touching, participation)

- **Learning disability** is a disorder which affects a child's ability to either adequately interpret what they see and hear, or to link the processed information from different parts of the brain.

OBSERVATIONAL

$\mathcal{M}$ETHODOLOGY

Ayo is a 2-year-old child, busy in his playful activity, surrounded by many colourful toys, a ball, some building blocks and a soft teddy bear. He tries to build a house with the blocks and is completely engrossed in his play; meanwhile, his mother comes out from the kitchen and holds him in arms, kisses him, appreciates his work and start helping him in making his home.

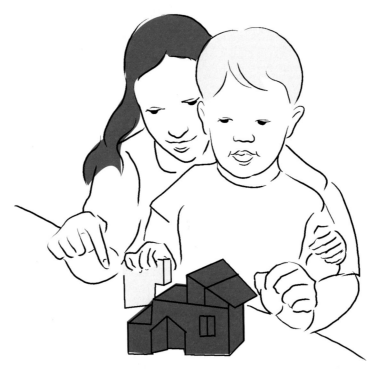

If we could see the miracle of a single flower clearly, our whole life would change.
-Buddha

Observation

Observation is gathering information from the real world by recognizing and noting facts or behaviour as they occur (1).

To observe is to take notice, to watch attentively or to focus on one particular aspect of the entire massive stimulus in the child's environment.

Observation is a technique, which everyone uses in his daily life. In casual situations, personal or situational biases may unconsciously influence the observational process. Formal records of casual observations are never kept and consequently it is just the memory that stores information. Whereas a scientific observation is done in a systematic and objective manner with careful record keeping that leads to valuable physical as well as behavioural information.

During early childhood development, aspects of a child's life and especially child-rearing practices can be observed.

Contextualization of Observation

Before using observation as a tool to collect information on any aspect, for instance about children and their environment, the objectives of the observation should be carefully planned, keeping in context the observation (2). Sometimes there is a great temptation to record every incidental matter as well, but recording irrelevant details or anything which is not the requirement for the study objective would be useless, and a waste of time, but at the same time, we cannot isolate an event from its context. If we are observing a child, it does not mean that we will not consider the happenings around him: rather, we are incorporating everything, which is part of his social environment. We are observing the caregiver – parent-child interactions, teacher-child interactions, the quality time they are giving to the child, the norms that depict their child rearing practices, and even current environmental changes that could potentially affect child development. Observation of the child in his/her context is an important strategy to assess the availability of stimulatory environment at home, at school, at the day care centre and even in the play area.

Process of Observation

The process of observation is based on following decisions that have to be made before starting the process:

Where to observe?

Observation can be carried out in various settings (3), but most commonly used settings are:

a)   Naturalistic Setting

b)   Structured Setting

a)   Naturalistic Setting

Observation of behaviour in a natural setting, without any attempt by the observer to intervene, is called naturalistic observation. This observation could be done at home, school or even at a playground. An observer in naturalistic setting acts as a passive recorder of what occurs, that is, the behaviour occurs ordinarily. It has not been arranged specifically for the purpose of recording behaviour (4).

An observer is attentively looking at 3-year-old Raja, who is watching his elder brothers playing cricket; whenever he approaches to join them in play, they refuse, as he is too young to play with them. Meanwhile his father arrives on the ground and Raja rushes towards him and tells him about the attitude of his brothers. The father scolds them and asks them to play with Raja. Now Raja seems happy because he is going to bat now.

Caregiver's observation

The caregiver's observation is very important regarding a child's holistic development. He/she is the person who remains in close contact with the child; any milestone achieved gives him/her the most pleasure while any observations of developmental delay urge her to take immediate consultation. Therefore, the role of the caregiver in terms of observing child health and development is considered vital. For instance, the caregiver can carefully observe and consult the nearest health facility if the child is not growing in height or weight.

The child's ability to show diverse emotions is a sign of healthy development. If the child is not exhibiting a range of emotions like joy, anger, sorrow and excitement persistently then it could be a sign for consultation with the health facility.

b)   Structured Setting

In this setting, the observer often intervenes in order to cause an event to occur or to set up a situation so that event can be more easily recorded (5). Observation can easily be done at the home or school settings.

Kiran is observing a 2-year-old child Kobi, who is playing in his courtyard. She takes out a ball from her bag, and gives it to the child to kick so that she can observe his psychomotor development.

What to observe?

The decision about what to observe can be further divided, so that the observer can either observe everything that a child does, or focus on specific behaviour; can observe the child alone or the immediate environment as well, such as responses of the people around the child, the quality of the home etc. This largely depends on the objectives of the observation (6). If one wants to investigate child-rearing practices then various related domains such as the quality time the caregiver is giving to the child, nutritional practices, hygiene practices etc. can be observed.

Asad is a 2 1/2-year-old child who is talking to his father. Asad seems happy his father is playing cricket with him; when the father throws a ball towards him, he tries excitedly to make a hit and laughs at his attempts whenever his father appreciates him by saying "you are a great batsman".

The observer notices that Najma, mother of 4-months old baby Akbar, is placing the head of the sleeping child on a mud block. The mother looks at the observer, who is curious to know about the practice, and asks if she knows the purpose of this block, the observer smiles and say "no", the mother smiles back and says that the block is used to make the child's head flat as a flat head is considered a symbol of beauty in her community.

Type of Observation

In observation, we cannot overlook the role of the observers, as it is the key determinant for getting information. Observation of behaviour by someone who plays an active and significant role in the situation or in the context in which behaviour is recorded is referred to as participant observation (7). Participant observation is further divided into two types:

a)   Undisguised Participant Observation

b)   Disguised Participant Observation

a)   Undisguised participant observation

In this type of observation the individuals who are being observed know that the observer is present for collecting information about their behaviour, which can be done in the assessment of children for the intellectual and developmental test, and even for anthropometric assessment.

An observer is assessing the psychomotor development of a 2 1/2-years-old child by asking the child to draw a circle on a sheet.

At this moment not only the child but also the caregivers are also aware that the child is being observed.

b)   Disguised participant observation

In this observation, those who are being observed do not know the observer's role.

Kiran, an observer, is sitting beside her co-worker who is busy interviewing the mother of a two year old child Kobi, the child is playing with clay toys in the courtyard near the stove: soon Kobi sees the

> *What we see depends mainly on what we look for.*
> -John Lubbock

> *An observer should always notice the home environment including the role of the caregivers.*

matchbox and tries to reach for it. His mother, who seems busy in the interview, sees of the child's action and rushes towards him shouting and scolding. She makes the child sit beside her so that she keep an eye on him.

The role of the observer is very important whether he acts in a disguised or undisguised manner. It is generally observed that people do not always behave in the way they ordinarily would when they know that their behaviour is being observed. If a caregiver knows that his/ her behaviour with the child is under observation, then they might start acting in a socially desirable way, to avoid negative evaluation by the observer.

How to record the observation?

Observations can be recorded in many different ways, from a comprehensive description of behaviours to quantifying certain behaviours (8,9). The most common and the easiest method of recording observation is the checklist.

The Checklist

This is used to record the presence or absence of something in the situation under observation. (1?) A further distinction can be made between static and action checklists.

a)   Static Checklist

A static checklist contains descriptions of the relatively permanent aspect of the subject or setting. Age and sex are examples of subject characteristics that are often noted. Similarly, features of the setting including time of the day, location, and whether or not other people are present can also be a part of a static checklist. **(See Appendix IV)**

b)   Action checklist

An action checklist is used to record the presence or absence of specific behaviours. **(See Appendix IV)**

Standardization of Observation

There are certain factors related to standardization of the observation, which must be considered; that is, the quality of the observation should be consistent.

a)   Duration of Observation

It is best to decide the time duration for the observation, which should be the same for all children under observation, in order to have uniform observation.

b)   Time

Standardization of time is another factor in collecting data for observation. The time must be the same in all cases in order to achieve standardized observation, e.g. it must be decided in advance whether to observe all children in the morning or in the evening.

c)   Number of observers

It is better to have a few trained observers for observation because having too many observers may lead to much variability in the observation, which definitely hampers the observation by making it inconsistent.

> *What is a weed? A plant whose virtues have not yet been discovered.*
> *-Ralph Waldo Emerson*

Conceptual understanding of some parent and child behaviour which is worthwhile to observe

1. Parenting Style
2. Reinforcement and punishment
3. Play

Parenting styles

Parenting is a concept of managing the growth and development of the child. Conventionally it has four domains (10)

- Control: clear provision of limit setting, disciplined
- Nurturance: food, cloth, shelter, warmth
- Maturity demands: expecting age appropriate behaviour
- Communication: responsive aspect of parent – child interaction

Based on these domains, parenting styles are generally divided into four types:

a) Authoritative Style: Parenting characterized by high levels of

- Control
- Nurturance
- Maturity demands
- Communication

Care giving is warm, responsive, and involved but gives freedom of expression and activity. Logical and practical limits are set and age appropriate mature behaviours are expected from children.

Undesirable behaviour of a child is dealt with affection, and reason behind his/her actions is inquired into and the behaviour expected from the child is communicated with logical reasoning.

b) Authoritarian style: Parenting characterized by high levels of

- Control and
- Maturity demands

In addition, low level of

- Nurturance
- Communication

Care giving is cold, unresponsive and rigid and relatively harsh punishment methods are used to discipline the children.

Undesirable behaviour of the child is dealt with punishment rather than trying to understand the child and talking with him/her about his conduct.

c) Permissive style:

Parenting characterized by high levels of

- Nurturance

In addition, low levels of

- Control
- Maturity demands
- Communication

A parent is an individual with short or long-term, primary care giving responsibility for a child.

- *Mother*
- *Father*
- *Grandparent*
- *Other relative*
- *Non-kinsperson*

such as a foster parent

Parent surrogate in an institutional setting

The hardest part of raising a child is teaching them to ride bicycles. A shaky child on a bicycle for the first time needs both support and freedom. The realization that this is what the child will always need can hit hard.

-Sloan Wilson

Care giving is lax and inconsistent with discipline and encouragement practices in response to free and untamed impulses of children.

Undesirable behaviour of the child is permitted; from time to time contradictory messages are given, e.g. by scolding on the act of aggression on one occasion, and considering the same deed as an act of bravery on another.

d) Neglecting style:

Parenting characterized by low levels of

- Control
- Nurturance
- Maturity demands
- Communication

Care giving is indifferent and neglectful with lack of focus on children's needs

Undesirable behaviour of the child is not attended to most of the time. Usually such parents have personal problems and are not able to handle them effectively, so are unable to attend to the child's needs.

Parenting style that is considered preferable for holistic child development is the authoritative style, while the rest of parenting styles inculcate some of those characteristics in a child's personality that badly affect his later functioning and adjustment within the environment. Authoritative parents with their responsiveness, warmth, clear limit setting and expectation of age appropriate behaviour turn out a child who is full of life, cheerful, social, self reliant, and achievement oriented. Consequently, such a child will be able to reach his/her optimal functioning in every domain of child development.

	Authoritative Style	*Authoritarian Style*	*Permissive Style*	*Neglecting Style*
Control	■	■		
Maturity demands	■	■		
Nurturance	■		■	
Communication	■			

High Level ■
Low Level

Reinforcement and punishment

Undesirable behaviour or temper tantrum of a child is usually dealt with punishment, which could be either physical or verbal: this in turn creates a communication gap between the child and caregiver. The child does not abandon that behaviour, but tries to avoid the source of punishment i.e. caregiver. Consequently, punishments badly affect the socio-emotional development of the child

Every act of a child has a specific reason; sometimes tantrums are a way of getting the caregiver's attention towards certain unmet needs, or poor understanding of the phenomenon, and sometimes they are the consequences of parenting style of the caregiver (11).

Instead of punishing the child, it is highly recommended to focus on building communication with him/her a strategy that not only helps the caregiver to understand the situation but also helps the child to express his views and build trust in the caregiver. It is also useful not to over-react when a child says "NO", because sometimes he or she may just say no without internalizing the instructions. The child actually means to be in control himself/herself and he will continue to say "NO" until he or she has thought it through, or

> ***Whenever I held my newborn baby in my arms, I used to think that what I said and did to him could have an influence not only on him but on all whom he met, not only for a day or a month or a year, but for all eternity - a very challenging and exciting thought for a mother.***
> ***-Rose Kennedy***

AUTHORITATIVE STYLE
Children are more likely to become confident, competent, independent, and affectionate persons.

> ***Punishment creates hostility in the child while communication and praise could create feelings of security and high self-esteem.***

PUNISHMENT
The practice of imposing something unpleasant on a wrongdoer

REINFORCEMENT
Act performed to strengthen approved behaviour

realizes the seriousness of the caregiver. Instead of dispensing punishment, answer the hidden challenge by repeating the request calmly and clearly.

Desirable behaviour should be rewarded, praised and noticed immediately when the child performs it. Such practice by the caregiver could increase the chances of occurrence of such behaviour in future, as the child would want to maintain the parent's approval.

Play

Play could be any activity, which the child enjoys; regardless of whether outdoor or indoor; it has elements of physical and mental activity (12).

A child tries to make sense of the physical world whether through exploration or imitation, and learns through active involvement, concentration, language development, curiosity and problem solving abilities. Therefore, in play, all mental, emotional and physical faculties of the child are involved and practiced which enhances his development. Play provides the opportunity to practice and strengthen new skills in a pleasurable way.

Playing with the sand can be a soothing sensory experience and provide a chance to the child to begin understanding about capacity and volume.

The role of a caregiver is very important with respect to a child's play, though it should not be an interfering role: rather it should be a participatory one. The child will gladly welcome parental suggestions if they are offered carefully and at the right time e.g.

If a child is playing with sand, show him/her how to make a house; he/she may or may not want to try, but do not interfere with his/her own plan.

Sometimes a caregiver can offer partnership, e.g. a child cannot play 'peek a boo', if nobody will play with him/her; similarly he or she cannot practice rolling and receiving a ball if no one else will play. Interactions and quality time by the caregiver or peers also enhances the socio-emotional development of the child.

Types of Play during Early Childhood

a)   **Sensory Motor Play:** by approximately age 1, children spend most of their playtime in exploration and manipulation of objects provided to them.
> *Infants place things in their mouths, or shake them and crawl along the floor.*

b)   **Constructive Play:** by approximately age 2, children bring into play objects in their surroundings to construct things with them. Resourcefulness of the environment helps them to play more enthusiastically.
> *Creating various shapes out of clay or with blocks*

c)   **First Pretend Play:** by approximately age 2, children also initiate pretend or make believe play
> *Taking care of dolls with pretended food, combing their hair with an imaginary comb, and pacifying them like a mother.*

Children are punished or rewarded by their
- *Parents*
- *Siblings*
- *Relatives*
- *Teachers*

PLAY
Act of occupying oneself in unrestrained, amusing interaction or recreation with people or things, which voluntarily or involuntarily leads to learning

---

Work and play are words used to describe the same thing under differing conditions.
-Mark Twain

You can discover more about a person in an hour of play than in a year of conversation.
-Plato

d) **Substitute Pretend Play:** by about age 2 to 3, children use items as a proxy for something different during play.

> *Feeding the doll with a pencil by naming or considering it a spoon*

e) **Socio-dramatic Play:** by age 3 to 5 or so, children begin to act in role-plays. This pretend play progresses from solitary to mutual play with other children. In play, a child always takes on more mature role than his age or routine behaviour.

> *Common childhood methods of play are "mother and baby", "teacher and student", "doctor and patient", "Marriage of dolls'.*

IMAGINARY COMPANION

It is regarded as a normal component of the development in children; it is no longer considered a sign of disturbance in a child

Significance of observational methodology in relation to early childhood development

Observation can be utilized in various settings

- Anthropometric assessment of the child
- Behavioural assessment of the caregiver and child
- Intellectual assessment of the child
- Capacity of the surroundings to provide stimulatory environment to the child i.e., home, school, day care centre and play area etc.

Summary

- **Observation of a child** is to watch attentively or to focus on specific aspect of the child behaviour in the context of his or her social environment.

- **The process of observation** involves identification of the setting: naturalistic vs. structured, decision about content of the observation, type of the observation: disguised vs. undisguised participant observation, and finally selection of the instrument for observation.

- **Standardization of Observation** can be achieved by maintaining consistency in duration of observation, time and number of observers

- **Parenting** is a concept of managing the growth and development of the child. Scientifically parenting is characterised by four domains; control, nurturance, maturity demands and communication with the child.

- **Parenting styles** are categorised into authoritative, authoritarian, permissive and neglecting styles based on different combinations of parenting domains.

- **Punishment** is the practice of imposing something unpleasant on a wrongdoer child for his or her undesirable behaviour.

- **Reinforcement** is the practice of rewarding a child for his or her desirable behaviour.

- **Play** is the act of occupying oneself in unrestrained, amusing interaction or recreation with people or things, which leads to voluntary or involuntary learning for the child.

- **Types of Play** during Early Childhood include *sensory motor play*: exploration and manipulation of objects provided to the child, *constructive play*: use of objects present in the surrounding to construct things, *first pretend play*: make believe play, *substitute pretend play*: use items as a proxy for something different during play, and *socio-dramatic play*: act in role-plays mutually with other children.

QUESTIONNAIRE

ᗷASED ᎥNTERVIEWS

*K*alsoom, a community health worker for communicable diseases, was on a routine visit to the community, when she met Rehana with a baby girl of about two months in her lap and a baby boy of one and a half years, in poor health, with her. Kalsoom began talking to her, and asked about any complaints of fever the two children may have had. The answer was yes, they did sometimes have bouts of fever. Before Kalsoom could ask another question, Rehana rushed to the stove to take care of cooking. As she returned, Kalsoom asked, "How high was the fever?" Rehana replied, "It was high, but only for a day." Kalsoom again asked, "Was it accompanied by any other health problem?"

Again Rehana had to leave the conversation to look after her mother–in–law, who was a patient of pulmonary tuberculosis. Rehana answered from the kitchen that the fever was accompanied by cough.

Kalsoom waited for Rehana to return, so that she could continue her questions in a more comfortable setting. Kalsoom asked another question: "Was the cough dry, or with sputum?" but before Rehana could answer, she had to go outside again, this time to milk the cow.

Kalsoom waited anxiously to complete the interview, but was helpless.

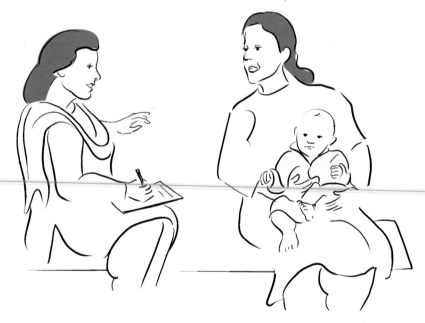

This was a very brief encounter between two individuals; one of whom was not fully satisfied because of the way in which the sequence of events proceeded, Kalsoom was unable to collect the information she needed.

Interview

The word interview implies a formal interaction between two or more people. Interviews vary in style and format. Interviews are particularly useful for getting the information and facts related to a specific aspect of knowledge, attitude, practices and status of an individual (1, 2).

Questionnaire

A questionnaire is a set of written questions used to collect data about opinions, attitudes, and knowledge (3, 4). It is perhaps the most ubiquitous method of obtaining information from people.

> *L*ife is essentially a question of values.
> -Meir Kahane

*O*btaining information from caregivers could be a very successful experience, provided the interviewer keep in mind cultural, socioeconomic and religious concerns during the process of interview.

QUESTIONNAIRE-BASED INTERVIEWS

The research interviewing technique allows person-to-person conversation that leads to information gathering regarding people's thoughts, feelings and behaviors specific only for the researcher's hypothesis. They are structured, based on predetermined questions and formal in nature.

IN-DEPTH INTERVIEWS

The research interviewing technique allows person to person discussion that leads to increased insight into people's thoughts, feelings and behaviors on respective issues. They are unstructured, based on guidelines and flexible in nature.

In Early Childhood Development (ECD) Research, face-to-face interview based on the questionnaire not only provides an opportunity to get direct information from the caregivers, but also provides an opportunity to educate them about the concepts and issues related to provision of a conducive environment for early childhood development in their households, as well as at community level.

Study Objectives

For the start of the training session for interviewers, it is obligatory to give a comprehensive account of the research project. An interviewer who is knowledgeable about the project can perform with greater confidence and get responses.

The comprehensive account of the ECD Project should at least include:

- A brief review of the situation analysis of the topic.
- Study objectives with their rationale.
- Methodology, especially eligibility criteria of selecting the caregiver of children in ECD Research.

It will help to justify each question's relevancy and specified format in the questionnaire.

Types of Questions Used in Interviews

The questions presented for interviews can be divided into two broad categories based on format and content:

On the Basis of Format

The two most important types of questions are close-ended and open-ended

Closed-ended Questions (Structured)

The interviewer of a study approached a family, with five children. The interviewer was upset as there were five children and she had to ask questions about the vaccination status of each child.
She asked: "Was the eldest child given any dose of vaccination?"
Mother replied: "No"
Interviewer repeated the same question for the second child, and the answer was the same. It was also negative for the other elder children; only for the youngest the answer was "Yes".
"How many injections were given?"
"Four"
"Was the schedule completed?"
"No, one injection was left to be given at the age of nine months."
The interviewer was very happy as she was expecting long and ambiguous answers, but whatever the responses were, they were very clear and short, giving clear understanding.

Structured questions are closely followed during the interview. The course of the interview is mostly predetermined, and little leeway is left for follow-up questions. A closed-ended question has fixed number of options, which allows the respondent to make a choice by choosing one of the listed options. Sufficient options are needed to fully cover the range of answers but these choices should not be so many that the distinction between them becomes blurred. Usually, five to ten possible answers per questions are considered reasonable. Examples of close-ended questions are True and False questions, Yes and No questions and multiple-choice questions *(See Appendix V, Q1.2, and Q2.2)*.

ADVANTAGES
- *Can quickly provide both quantitative and/or qualitative data*
- *Less resource dependent*

DISADVANTAGES
- *Questions and response options are fixed*
- *Requires good communication skills of the interviewer as well as interviewee*

A good questionnaire should comprehensively encompass the specific objectives of the research study.

The same questions with same response options will be asked of every respondent. Closed questions can usually be answered quickly, allowing the interviewer to get a lot of information quickly.

	CLOSE ENDED	OPEN ENDED
Limited response options		
Ease of administration		
Cost effectiveness of the information		
Interpretation influenced by researcher's perspective		

Increase	
Decrease	

Open-Ended Questions (Semi-Structured)

Sajida, an LHW, on her third visit to her community asked Amina: "What feed should be given to a child who reaches the age of weaning?" Amina replied with a detailed account of various food types available or practiced in that community such as: rice with milk, bread in gravy, boiled eggs, fruit in small pieces, prepared juices, meat with vegetables... (Sajida thought about her answer; it was open like a continuous flow of water from the pipe of tube well in her village!)

The open-ended questions are based on written lists of questions or topics that need to be covered in a particular order. These lists are called interview guides.

Open format questions are those that have no predetermined set of responses, and the participant is free to answer i.e., they don't select "yes" or "no" or provide a numeric rating, etc. The same open-ended questions are asked of all interviewees, who should think of their own responses and describe them in their own words *(See Appendix V, Q 2.1)*.

Open format questions are good for soliciting subjective data or when the range of responses is not clearly available.

On the Basis of Contents

Usually five kinds of questions are presented to the respondent based on the content of the questions :

a)   *Practice* - about what a person has done or is doing
       At what age did you start to wean your child?

b)   *Attitude* - about what a person thinks about a topic
       What do you think about weaning practices in your community?

c)   *Knowledge* – about what information a person has regarding a topic
       What is the appropriate age to start weaning the baby?

d)   *Sensory* - about what people have seen, touched, heard, tasted or smelt.
       What variety of taste have you introduced during the first month of weaning?
       In what kind of environment will you feed your baby?

e)   *Demographic* – This information provides information about the general characteristics of an individual such as age, gender, marital status, education, etc.

What is the age of your baby?

Format of the Questionnaire

The interview schedule in a sample survey is not a simple list of questions; it is a multi-faceted instrument to collect data. The questionnaire can be divided into three main parts: the informed consent, the face sheet and the body.

Informed Consent (See Appendix VI)

It is each individual's autonomy regarding the decision of complete, partial or no involvement in the interview process (5, 6).

The fundamental requirement of informed consent is agreement on a series of statements presented by interviewer to the respondent.

a) **Description of the research project**
This should include the purpose of the research, reason the subject is being asked to participate, amount of time expected of the subject, and a simplified description of the methodology, keeping in mind the comprehension requirements of the respondent such as language, terminologies etc.

b) **Statement of voluntary participation**
There will be no penalty because of refusal to participate, and the subjects can discontinue participation at any time without penalty. The caregiver must never be coerced to participate in the research.

c) **Description of any benefits and foreseeable discomforts**
Benefit means direct benefits (financial remuneration or other compensation), not just "adding to the body of knowledge" in the field of ECD. If there is any discomfort, the respondent should be informed about the measures that the researcher is taking to minimize them.

d) **Statement concerning confidentiality**
Collected information will be only utilized to reach a generalized conclusion about the study population; no reference should ever be made about the individual respondent.

e) **Contact information**
The informed consent must contain the complete address and telephone number of the investigator, in order to understand his/her rights or the results during the research process.

Face Sheet and Body of the Questionnaire (See Appendix-V and VII)

This portion of the questionnaire includes :
- Actual questions to be asked
- Answer categories
- Code numbers assigned to each question and answer category
- Instructions to the interviewer regarding questioning

INFORMED CONSENT
ECD Research involving children requires the written consent of the primary caregiver.

ECD REINFORCEMENTS
Informed Consent
Ethically, informed consent must be obtained virtually from every participant of the ECD project.

Ideally, a copy of the informed consent should be given to the respondent.

a) Response Cards

When the structured response categories are many and difficult to understand, or to retain in one's memory, then it is advisable to use a response card. This helps the respondent to look at all the choices before giving any answer. For the illiterate respondent, response cards with pictorial instead of written options are advised.

b) Skip Pattern

In many surveys, the interview schedule contains more questions than are asked of any one respondent, because it is often necessary to ask one question before knowing whether other questions apply to the particular respondent. The pattern these questions follow is referred to as the skip pattern. It is important that the format clearly show the alternative routes to follow in the sequence of questions.

Sampling

To select an eligible respondent, an interviewer has to sample the population according to the following protocol (7):

Mapping and Framing of the Area (See Appendix-VIII)

The entire area of the community (study population, on which study is being conducted) is mapped out geographically. This numbering task is carried out in a way that all villages or blocks of a locality, streets and houses are clearly demarcated on a map by making a list of demographic information of all eligible children in the study area.

Eligible candidates

Eligibility of a respondent depends on the objectives of a study.

For a study of determining the practices of childcare (<3 years) the element here is an eligible child less than three years old and a resident of the Mari Community. After mapping of the Mari community and making a sampling frame of the area. Below 3 years children are identified in these households. As this age group is not able to respond to the questions, therefore, the caregivers of these children are recruited for interviews. Consequently, caregivers are the respondents in this type of study.

When there is more than one eligible candidate in one household then one of them is selected randomly.

Selection of Respondents

We can sample the respondent and households through two basic strategies.

a) Simple Random Sampling

In this strategy, every member element in the study population can be potentially sampled .

A numbered list will be prepared of all the children below the age of three living in the area. At the same time the same number of small pieces of paper will be arranged, on which the number of every child will be written. For example, if there are 120 children and out of them, a sample of 30 is to be drawn, then 120 pieces of paper will be prepared and on them, the child number from 1-120 will be written. These papers will be closed and thoroughly mixed. One piece of paper will then be picked up randomly at a time until the desired number of 30 children are selected for the interview.

This method has no personal influence of the researcher on the selection of the participants, either consciously or unconsciously.

SAMPLING UNITS
Individual 0-6 year old child of the defined population, whose characteristics are to be measured.

SAMPLING FRAME
List or map that identifies every 0-6 year old child (sampling unit) in the defined population. Such a list is needed so that every individual child of the population can be identified unambiguously.

b) Systematic Sampling

In this strategy, the first step is estimation of the number of respondents (children) required out of the total population . Divide the total number of children (e.g.120) by the required sample of the children (e.g.30) in the population, the number obtained after division is called the sampling interval. Select first child randomly between one and four (the sampling interval) from the sampling frame, for example, which comes out to be three. The child on number three is selected for interview. For the second child four is added to three (sampling interval) and for the third child four is added to seven (sampling interval) and so on until all the 30 children are selected.

Framework of Children < 3 years

1 2 |3| 4 5 6 |7| 8 9 10 |11| ....

Pre-testing

Pre-testing is necessary before administering an ECD Research Questionnaire finally in the field (8). In pre-testing the following points are assessed:

Try the questionnaire on a similar but not the same community, on which final data will be collected to identify potential weaknesses and difficulties. Write notes to clarify any scratching, ensure pages are numbered, make a note of all the observations, during an interview for instance.

- Did any question have element of threat to the interviewee?
- Time consumption per questionnaire and per specific area/unit of study population?
- Was there any ambiguity in the questions or response?

General Guidelines for Conducting Interviews

There are some points that are important to consider before and during the interview process (9);

Preparation for Interview

Setting / Environment

- Avoid loud lights or noises; ensure the interviewee is comfortable (you might ask them if they are), etc. Often, they may feel more comfortable at their own places of work or homes.
- Provide informed consent to the respondent.
- Indicate the time required for the interview.
- Ask them if they have any questions before the interview.

Interview

- Ask one question at a time.
- Attempt to remain as neutral as possible.
- Encourage responses with occasional nods of the head, "uh huh"s, etc.
- Provide transition between major topics,
  "We've been talking about eating habits of the child, and now I'd like to move on to the activity pattern of your child"
- Do not lose control of the interview. This can occur when respondents stray to another topic, take so long to answer a question that time begins to run out, or even begin asking questions of the interviewer.

> *To do a really good interview, you have to be truly interested in the person.*
> -Daisy Fuentes

> *If you're doing an interview, you need conversational tension. After you talk to them, you're not going to have a relationship with them, they're not going to like you, they're not going to be your friend.*
> -Chuck Klosterman

- Avoid personal enquiries.
- An interviewer should be well versed in the local language
- A standard approach should be maintained for all respondents with regard to prompting and total time spent in an interview.

Handling of Refusals

Refusals could be partial and or complete. At times, it is not refusals but non-availability of the respondent.

a) Partial

Sometime respondents do not clearly say 'No', but they do not respond to some of the questions. This non-response could be due to the inappropriate approach of the interviewer, lack of comprehension, or cultural sensitivity of the topic. The interviewer should politely inquire into the reason for the partial refusal and try to make changes to the interviewee's satisfaction. If the interviewee persists in giving the same type of response, his/her, decision should be respected.

b) Complete

In our culture/village norms, the probability of refusal is less when interviewer establishes personal contact rather than requests the appointment through phone or letter.

The fact sheet of these individuals should be completely filled if they refuse to give a formal interview inorder to assess during analysis, whether non-respondent have characteristics as compared to those who respond or are partially non-respondent.

c) Non-availability

Due to time constraints, some respondents may respond negatively, especially when there is no prior contact. At this point, the best option is to set an appointment for some other time . When respondents are not available for an introductory as well as follow up visit, the best option is to wait for the potential respondent if he/she is expected back soon, leave a message for the respondent with the family members, pointing out the importance of her/his inclusion in the interviews.

Quality Control of Data
a) The Need for Quality Control

The data collection phase of a study is a challenging job. The appropriate procedures for monitoring are deficient in quality, then problems with missing and/or erroneous data may occur (10).

b) Inaccurate or Imprecise Data

When more than one person collect data without any check, then such problems are likely to arise that seriously affect the results. This happens when one of the team members applies a consistently wrong technique to measurement. The situation becomes very grave when errors in the data cannot be detected after the fact. This is no exception even in cases where the investigator is working alone on a small study. The only practical solution is to develop a systematic quality control program.

c) Quality Control of Data Management

- At the completion of an interview, the interviewer should have a quick review and confirm the completion of the form.
- Conduct periodic surprise checks by field supervisors.
- Carry out regular editing of the questionnaire after the interview with thorough review of the form

Quality questions create a quality life. Successful people ask better questions, and as a result, they get better answers.
-Anthony Robbins

Quality is never an accident; it is always the result of intelligent effort.
-John Ruskin

and validation of responses with some similarities.

- After completion and editing of the questionnaire, coding of the different responses to questions is done before data entry.

- Responses of potentially close-ended questions should be pre-coded. If it is possible, "don't know" and "missing information" responses should contain a code i.e. "98" and "99" respectively. The same numeric code should be followed throughout the questionnaire.

- On the other hand, responses to open ended questions are often coded after completion of the interview. To ensure and maintain consistency and reliability, a comprehensive coding manual should be prepared.

Summary

- *A Questionnaire* is a set of written questions used to collect data about opinions, attitudes, and knowledge from a person of interest.

- *Questionnaire based interview* is a research interviewing technique which allows person-to-person formal conversation leading to information gathering regarding thoughts, feelings and behaviours of the respondent.

- *Questions* can be classified on the basis of their format into Close-ended and Open –ended, while on the basis of their content they can be categorized into Knowledge, Attitude, Practice, Sensory and Demographic.

- *Informed Consent* is each respondent's autonomy regarding the decision of complete, partial or no involvement in the interview process. ECD Research involving older children requires the written consent of the primary caregiver.

- *A Questionnaire consists* of informed consent, face sheet and the body of the questionnaire.

- *Sampling* is a process of selection of study respondents, from among all eligible in the population as per prescribed protocol.

- *Pre-testing* is the trial of the questionnaire on a similar but not the same community on which final data will be collected. Pre-testing is used to identify potential weaknesses and difficulties, especially ambiguity and sensitivity of specific questions, and time consumption.

- *Standardized approach* should be maintained for all respondents especially with regard to interview setting, language, prompting and total time spent in an interview.

- *Quality Control* of data from questionnaires can be achieved by developing the appropriate mechanism to monitor the interview process, and after regular checking of the questionnaire to rectify the problems with missing and erroneous information.

> *There is nothing to fear except the persistent refusal to find out the truth, the persistent refusal to analyze the causes of happenings.*
> -Dorothy Thompson

focus group

DISCUSSION

In a room, a group of women are seated discussing various topics. Some are discussing their children's health, some domestic work, and some are chatting on community events. However, as their conversation is not focused on one topic, we cannot conclude anything from it. Then a woman from the group asks, "What is the purpose of swaddling a child?" Answers start coming from different directions; some say it strengthens the muscles, some say that the child can sleep well…This is how the conversation turns to a particular direction; the group starts talking about the issue in relation to early childhood development.

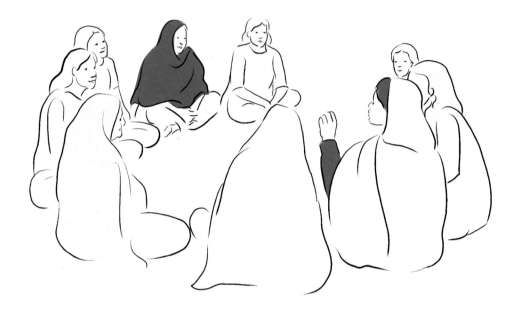

FOCUS GROUP DISCUSSION
Carefully planned discussion designed to obtain perceptions in a defined area of interest in a permissive and non-threatening environment moderated by a facilitator

GENERAL DISCUSSION
Casual dialogue among people on any topic without any moderation by a facilitator or without following any ground rules.

GROUP INTERVIEWING
Emphasis is on interviewing a number of people at the same time, based on questions from the researcher and specific responses from each member of the group.

FOCUS GROUP DISCUSSION
Emphasis is on interaction within the group, based on topics that are assigned by the researcher.

Focus Group Discussion

Focus Group Discussion (FGD) is a method of gathering qualitative information, which is aimed at gaining information about a specific issue through group interaction, and with the active participation of a facilitator (1, 2). As opposed to a general interview, the primary goal of a focus group discussion is to create an environment where people are encouraged to talk to one another, asking questions, responding, exchanging and narrating experiences and points of view on a selected topic. Focus group discussions can help explore how and why people behave as they do in their own words, to understand their emotional reaction to a certain issue, or to understand the way they see the world. In short, it is a method of obtaining a range of opinions from people about a specific topic of interest.

Preparation for a Focus Group Discussion

On the surface, conducting a focus group discussion may appear to be an easy process; however, in reality it requires a great deal of preparation in order to facilitate a successful focus group discussion (3, 4, 5). Some preparatory steps are required before actually conducting a focus group discussion in the field:

The first step in preparing to conduct focus group discussions is to develop a set of guidelines. The guidelines must include:

a) Objectives for conducting focus group discussion:
To understand the need for conducting a focus group discussion, and obtain a specific type of information from the participants.

"The purpose of conducting these focus group discussions is to identify factors related to child rearing

practices that are conducive to the learning ability of a child."

b) Target Groups:

It is important to identify a group of people with whom the research team would like to conduct the focus group discussions.

> *For a research topic related to early childhood development, possible target groups could include those that play the role of caregivers, i.e. mothers, fathers, adolescent siblings, school teachers etc.*

The number of groups required for focused discussions depends upon the number of different subgroups or distinct population segments existing in the target population. If the target population consists of caregivers of 0-6 year old child , then at least one focus group discussion is required with each type of caregiver: mother, fathers, siblings, relatives, teachers etc.

c) Group Size:

It is generally recommended that a group consist of 6 to 12 persons, in order to provide enough room for participants to participate in the ongoing discussion. Fewer than 6 participants may provide an insufficient number for a stimulating dialogue, and more than 12 may prove difficult to facilitate; such a large group may not provide an opportunity for all participants to express their points of view.

d) Composition of the Group:

The selection of the group is extremely important. The general preference is for a group, which is homogenous in terms of common denominators such as age, gender, residence or socio-economic status (6). Lack of homogeneity in circumstances may lead to difficulty in facilitating a group.

> *If the discussion concerns the issues of participants from a lower socio-economic class in the focus group, the presence of participants from a higher socio- economic class could inhibit the true expression of participants belonging to the lower socio-economic class.*

Participants in a focus group discussion should have a common background; however, it is preferable that they have no acquaintance with each other. This will ensure open discussion and free sharing of opinions among participants.

e) Duration:

Usually focus group discussions last about 1.5 to 2 hours; however, this depends on the nature of the topic and the number of the participants.

f) Recording Information:

It is important to identify the method by which information will be recorded during the focus group discussion. The role of a Note-taker and an Observer are significant in this respect. A note-taker records the entire discussion. The role of a note-taker in a focus group discussion is important, as in many cases participants may not feel comfortable in speaking when they know their voices are being recorded on tape. The observer notes the non-verbal communication and the group dynamics. Information provided by an observer will assist in the analysis of the discussion.

g) Discussion Guidelines:

Finally, the most important element in a focus group guideline is the set of questions, which help facilitate participants, invite them to share their views as fully as possible, share information with them and guide

> *If we knew what we were doing, it wouldn't be called research, would it?*
> *-Albert Einstein*

FOCUS GROUP DISCUSSION
Focuses on words and observations to express reality and attempts to describe people in usual situations.

QUESTIONING FORMAT
- *Open ended*

PATTERN
- *More general to the more specific;*
- *Questions of greater importance should be placed early.*

NUMBER
- *Focused discussion should not include more than six to eight questions.*

"Reason and free inquiry are the only effectual agents against error.
-Thomas Jefferson"

them towards sharing information related to the topic.

Given below are some examples from a discussion guide related to prevailing child rearing practices of children aged between 0 to 6 years.

- *Who are the caregivers of children aged between 0 to 6 years?*
- *What activities do you have with your child?*

Process of Focus Group Discussion

a) Planning:

Before conducting a focus group discussion, it is important that the entire sequence of how the focus group discussion will be conducted is reviewed in detail with all team members. The role of the facilitator is the key in actually conducting the discussion and he/she must have proper training in conducting a focus group discussion

ESSENTIAL SKILLS OF THE FOCUS GROUP DISCUSSION FACILITATOR

Leadership skills
- *Mental alertness*
- *Analytical ability*
- *Proficiency in communication*
- *Balance of control and non-directive appoach i.e. allowing the discussion to lead in new directions as long as the subject matter is pertinent.*

Interpersonal skills
- *Quick rapport building*
- *Attentive Listening*
- *Non-reactive*
- *Encouraging group members to express their views.*
- *Never expressing personal opinions or making judgments.*

Managerial Skills
- *Time management.*
- *Memorising the questioning pattern.*
- *Creating a relaxed and informal atmosphere.*
- *Free from anxieties and mental pressures.*

A way to ensure that the focus group discussion runs smoothly is to conduct a test focus group discussion among the research team which will allow for an opportunity to make changes where needed, and to practice using the guidelines.

b) Welcome:

Facilitator thanks the participants for taking the time out to attend the focus group.

c) Introduction of the team:

When a facilitator greets the participants and introduces the team, no professional titles such as Doctor or Engineer should be used. Designations generally make participants in small community settings feel inferior and insecure; therefore, using first names is a better and more advisable option.

d) Purpose of focus group discussion:

After the introduction, the facilitator shares the purpose of the focus group:

> "We are from an organization (name of the organization) and working on a topic related to early childhood development; we want to see the factors related to child rearing practices that are conducive to the learning ability of a child."

e) Introduction of the participants:

This is usually done through an icebreaker that is an activity, which allows the group to feel more comfortable in each other's presence and in expressing themselves. In addition, the demographics of the participants that is name, age, educational background etc. should be recorded in the proceedings of focus group discussion's by the note-taker.

f) Informed Consent:

Refer to the chapter on Questionnaire-Based Interviews.

g) Ground Rules:

Before starting the discussion it is important to stress that there are no right or wrong answers and that everyone's participation is valued. In addition, it is also a good idea to suggest some norms for the discussion. These can be set in collaboration with the participants, for example:

- One should avoid interrupting if someone is sharing his/her views
- Everyone should have an opportunity to share their opinion
- If you would like to speak, raise your hand
- Speak one at a time

The aim of an argument or discussion should not be victory, but progress.
-Joseph Joubert

h) The Discussion:

Initially in the warm up session, the facilitator begins by asking general questions *(for example, who usually takes care of the child?)* moving to more specific questions as the discussion gets underway. While discussing it is important that the facilitator communicate genuine interest in the individual responses and questions. The facilitator should not be judgemental about the discussion. Once the participants begin to interact, it is frequently necessary for the facilitator to probe further.

> *Facilitator: What activities do you have with your child?*
> *Participant: We are busy with our child throughout the day.*
> *Facilitator now probes and asks Right; let me ask you to elaborate a little bit.*
> *Participant: I feed my child, talk with him, play with him....*

Hence, a probe can be used to clarify the concepts and responses, and to get a genuine and complete answer. For probing, it is not always necessary to go for a direct question; even a facilitator's silence or perhaps occasional nodding can encourage the group to continue on their own.

ETHICAL ISSUES
Participants: encouraged to maintain confidentiality of the contents of the discussion

Researchers: responsible for maintaining anonymity of information from the discussion

i) Conclusion:

As the discussion reaches its end, it is important that the facilitator does not allow the discussion to extend beyond the scheduled time. Before the end, the facilitator can summarize the main points of the discussion and allow the participants to express their final thought on the focus group in general and then thank the participants.

Types of focus group discussions

Based on their content, focus group discussions can be categorized into two types.

Exploratory focus groups

Forum of discussions regarding the caregiver's perception, understanding or even needs regarding child development.

Experiential focus groups

Forum of discussions regarding caregiver's experiences, observation or even motivation level for potentials and challenges regarding child development.

Experiential focus groups can be further explained with the understanding of positive experience in child development.

Positive Experiences

Care-giving practices and skills can result in both positive as well as negative child developmental outcomes. It is always meaningful to explore actively the causes and mechanism, of relatively positive experiences rather than assuming the desirable developmental status as just an outcome of absence of negative child caring practices. This shift-of-thinking paradigm is important for creating awareness about that which is achievable within the limited resources available at family and community level. In this context, an innovative use of experiential focus groups can be very helpful in identifying, discussing and motivating the caregiver to adopt positive child rearing practices.

Positive Deviance

Positive deviance describes a single or a set of child rearing practices that result in more than the expected growth and developmental status of the child: however, these practices are generally limited to only a few families in the community (7).

DEVIANCE
Change from the normal or usual

POSITIVE DEVIANCE
Constructive deviation from the normal child rearing practices of the caregiver, resulting in more than expected growth and developmental status of the child

POSITIVE DEVIANT
Caregiver who is able to utilize more effectively existing resources in the environment for the betterment of the child

At family level, significant variation exists in the caregiver's capacity, skills, care, nurturance and expression of warmth irrespective of their soaring levels of love and sincerity. At community level, despite the shared perspective of teachers or education personnel, handling the needs of a child differ from person to person. However, some caregivers exhibit a high level of skill or technology in child rearing irrespective of their socioeconomic status, resulting in better development of their children.

Timely positive gain in a child's growth and development has not only short-term implications but also

ECD REINFORCEMENTS
Explore the causes and mechanism of relatively positive experiences rather than assuming the desirable developmental status as just an outcome of absence of negative child caring practices.

Reasons for child's growth and developmental success should be explored more than failure.

MATERNAL TECHNOLOGY
Refers to practices, behaviours and beliefs of the caregiver related to
- *Handling of food and water*
- *Feeding pattern*
- *Personal hygiene*
- *Child care and interaction*
- *Sensory stimulation*
- *Safety and security*

results in achievement of enduring abilities of physical, psychological and emotional strengths. During adulthood, such children are better able to cope with life's stresses, and can accommodate in a new environment with relative ease. These individuals are able to persistently struggle in the face of unfavourable conditions; they try to deal constructively with day-to-day challenges. Despite adverse experiences, these traits allow a person to survive and flourish socially as well as economically. Thus better care giving in the early years not only makes them less susceptible to risk in later life, but enables them to spring back and achieve their life goals even in the face of unfavourable circumstances.

It is a fact that millions of children in developing countries are living in a considerably compromised state, with gross deficiencies in nutrition, care and social environment. It is understandable that they will never be able to achieve their physical, emotional and intellectual potential, and will be caught in a vicious cycle of vulnerability throughout their lives.

However, we sometimes observe a small proportion of well-nourished and psychologically and socio-emotionally well-developed children in resource-scarce families and communities. This pattern of growth gives hope that it is still possible to identify certain child-caring practices that resulted in positive child developmental outcomes despite poverty and limited resources. In these circumstances, identification of positive deviance in families or communities provides us with a reason to implement community-based intervention, and give content and strategy based on that successful behaviour.

Interventions based on positive deviance are primarily related to change in the behaviour of the caregiver based on examples existing in the neighbourhood and community. This model behaviour is easily followed by them because they can identify with the problem, become positively deviant and look forward to a successful outcome. It thus becomes easy to understand that such behaviours are possible with the same resources and within the same environment. In addition, positive deviants can themselves take on the role of advocates of such action; this will be more reassuring and believable to the community, because one of their own members is communicating and suggesting to them the solutions to child development challenges.

The basic assumption about positive deviant caregivers is that they have the same resources as those accessible to their neighbours and community. However, they are distinguishable in certain care-giving practices, beliefs and child outcomes. This difference of practice and outcome could be at any level i.e. physical, socio-emotional or intellectual.

Positive Deviance Inquiry for ECD

Formally, positive deviants can be recognized by conducting community wide baseline situation analysis, followed by identification of positive deviance, concept formation, behaviours trial, and community wide implementation of the intervention of conducive practices for child development.

Informally, community or neighbourhoods take this initiative with the help of the tool of experiential focus groups. A local committee can be formed with the agenda of

- Discussion of the issues and challenges for ECD
- Identification of positive deviants
- Systematic inquiry of the reasons for successful children, for identification of distinctive practices and attitudes of the positive deviants in the community
  - Family level: caregiver characteristics (workload, physical health, reproductive history), maternal technology, social support system, and priorities in relation to expenditure on nutrition, health and education. etc.

VULNERABLE
Some children develop into psychologically ailing adults due to poor nurturing or traumatic early circumstances.

RESILIENT
Some children develop into psychologically healthy adults despite poor nurturing or traumatic early circumstances.

Better child growth and development is not necessarily correlated with economic status.

Positive Deviance does not guarantee an ideal outcome: but it does mean relatively better growth and development of the child.

Despite sharing the same environment caregivers sometimes differ from their contemporaries with respect to their acceptability of
- *Novel ideas*
- *New value systems*
- *Modern lifestyles*

- Community level: socioeconomic characteristics, availability and utility pattern of health, childcare centres, education and recreational resources. etc.
- Communication about the successful behaviours
- Development of feasible strategies on the basis of identified behavioural patterns
- At the same forum, motivate the community to put into practice the above strategies.

The community can accomplish this agenda through innovative application of experiential focus groups. In addition, even a circle of families can attempt this exercise of identifying successful behaviours and adapting them.

Positive Deviance and Sustainability

During the ECD program implementation, sometimes the community receives financial and material support from their collaborative development organizations. After depletion of those resources and ends of collaboration, the community usually regains its pre-program status. However,

ECD REINFORCEMENTS
Positive deviance implemented through experiential focus groups guarantees that resources already exist in the community; solutions of ECD challenges are identified, developed and implemented by the community. This control over conceptualization and resources is a vital motivation in the evolution and sustainability of ECD endeavours by the community.

ECD REINFORCEMENTS
Positive deviance implemented through experiential focus groups guarantees that resources already exist in the community; solutions of ECD challenges are identified, developed and implemented by the community. This control over conceptualization and resources is a vital motivation in the evolution and sustainability of ECD endeavours by the community.

Significance of Focus Group Discussions for Early Childhood Development

Focus group discussions have been conducted in multiple disciplines/fields as a useful form of conducting qualitative research. The utility of this method in the area of early childhood development is also significant.

- They can help explain the relationship between the stimulus and the effect.
  Contouring the head of a child is a common practice in certain communities and focus group discussions have been used to understand the reasoning and consequences of the practice.

- Focus group discussion's can also assist in the design of certain intervention strategies in relation to early childhood development, through understanding the needs of community members and providing a forum for community participation from the outset of the process.

- Focus group discussions can also assist in exploring the motivation level of a community when bringing change in issues related to early childhood development.

- Focus group discussions can also have a dual objective of creating awareness in community members on matters that may be beneficial for their child.
  "In the case of a focus group discussion on childhood vaccination, by the end of the discussion participants realize that vaccination is an essential requirement for the wellbeing of a child."

Summary

- A **focus group discussion** (FGD) is an organized dialogue by a facilitator, with a selected group of representatives comprising individuals from the target population to gain information about their knowledge, attitude, perceptions and experiences on a theme of interest.

- **General discussion** is casual dialogue among people on any topic without any moderation by a facilitator, or without any ground rules. Instead of interaction, in **Group interviewing** the emphasis is on interviewing a number of people at the same time, based on questions from the researcher and specific responses from each member of the group.

- **Guidelines** for conduct of the focus group discussion include conceptualization of the objectives of the proposed discussion, consideration of the target groups, number and composition of participants, defining role of a note-taker and observer for recording information, and a set of questions and directions for probing.

- **Steps** for conducting a focus group discussion include planning logistics, defining the role of facilitator and dry run of the sequence. A focus group discussion should start with the welcome address, introduction of the host as well as participants, followed by description of the purpose of the focus group discussion, informed consent of participants and the setting of ground rules by the facilitator. Discussion on the given objectives should be concluded with a summarization of the salient discussion points and thanks to the participants.

- **Exploratory focus groups discussions** are conducted to explore the caregiver's perception, understanding or even needs regarding child development. **Experiential focus groups discussions** explore the caregiver's experiences, observation or even motivation level for potentials and challenges regarding child development

- **Positive Deviance** is a departure from the normal or routine child rearing practices of the caregiver, resulting in more than expected growth and developmental status of the child.

- **Formal positive deviance inquiry** is conducted by recognition of positive deviants through community wide baseline situation analysis, concept formation, behaviours trial and community wide implementation of the intervention of conducive practices for child development.

- **Informal positive deviance inquiry** is conducted by the initiative of neighbourhoods with the help of experiential focus groups discussion for the issues and challenges for ECD, identification of positive deviants, and distinguishing practices and attitudes of positive deviants, followed by communication of the successful behaviours to the community, to motivate them to follow those practices and behaviours.

> *The men of experiment are like the ant, they only collect and use; the reasoners resemble spiders, who make cobwebs out of their own substance. But the bee takes the middle course: it gathers its material from the flowers of the garden and field, but transforms and digests it by a power of its own.*
> -Francis Bacon

chapter nine

COMMUNICATION

Basic Components of Communication
Sender
Receiver
Message
Feedback

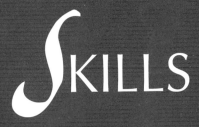

SKILLS

Factors Enabling Effective Communication

Types of Communication
Verbal communication
Nonverbal Communication

Domains of Communication
Language
Paralinguistic features
Body language
Facial expressions
Eye contact
Body space and proximity
Touch
Physical appearance

Communication Skills in Interviews
Considerations for a good speaker
Considerations for a good listener

Guidelines for Communication Skills with Respect to Interviewer
Beginning the interview
The main part of the interview
Ending the interview

Guidelines for Communication skills for various target groups in relation to ECD
Communicating with Infants (0 to 18 months)
Communicating with Toddlers (18 months to 3 years)
Communication with children (3 to 6 years)
Communication with Caregivers

Counselling in the Context of ECD
The Techniques
Prescriptive Counselling
Informative Counselling
Counselling Process
Counselling Skills

Non-Verbal Skills

Verbal Skills

Summary

> *Grown-ups never understand anything for themselves, and it is tiresome for children to be always and forever explaining things to them.*
> -Saint-Exupéry

A 2-year-old child is sitting on the floor playing with his toy, when suddenly the child's elder brother comes towards him and snatches the toy away. The child starts to cry. Meanwhile, the child's mother comes and tries to calm the boy down by giving him another toy, but he throws that away and asks for the toy he was playing with earlier. The mother becomes angry and slaps the child, and he starts to cry loudly. The mother takes the child in her lap and starts patting him on his back: he becomes quiet, and starts to play with his mother.

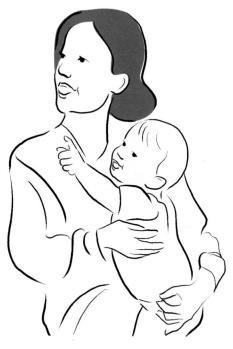

Communication means the sharing of thoughts, either in a verbal or non-verbal way

Communication can be defined as "the act of imparting or transmitting ideas, information." Communication is a complex, dynamic process in which the participants simultaneously create and share meaning in an interaction. The goal is the achievement of common understanding of the message sent and received. It is a process which enables us to establish interpersonal relationships (1).

The human skills required to complete the process of communication are referred to as Communication Skills, and are equally applicable for both the sender and receiver of the message.

Basic Components of Communication

It consists of a sender, a receiver, message and feedback, set within a particular context (2, 3).

Sender

The Sender is a person who conveys a particular message. It could be conscious but could be beyond the direct awareness of the sender. The sender is the source of information and initiator of the communication process. The sender sends the message by putting it into words, gestures and facial expressions.

Receiver

The Receiver is a person who receives the message and comprehends its meaning. The receiver may register what was intended to be sent, but often receives more as well, especially the unconscious component.

Message

The Message is the content of the communication, which is to be sent from one person to another person. The message can be categorized based on its level in the communication.

Feedback

The feedback is the integral part of the communication process whereby the sender and receiver exchange information, clarify information through verbal and non-verbal communication, and the receiver responds to the sender. The non-verbal examples include smiling, nodding of head, and acknowledgement.

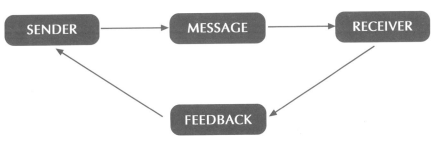

Basic Components of Communication with Feedback

Factors Enabling Effective Communication

Sender

- Social and cultural similitude between sender and receiver
- Positive attitude of the sender
- Sufficient emphasis by the sender
- Sender should convey the message confidently and explicitly
- Sender should modify the language of message according to the educational and social background of the receiver

Receiver

- Receptiveness of receiver
- Understanding and memory

Message

- Lengthy messages are usually confusing and not received well, so for education regarding early childhood development the message should be short, precise and direct.

Types of Communication

There are two main types of communication (4):

Verbal communication:

This system of communication includes spoken words to convey the message.

Non-verbal Communication:

This system of communication includes facial expression, body movements, and gestures, commonly referred to as body language or nonverbal communication.

LEVELS OF MESSAGES
The sent message: intended meaning of the sender.

The transmitted message: specified in terms of the medium used.

The received message: meaning perceived by the recipient.

FEEDBACK
Response by a receiver to the sender's message, either verbally or non-verbally or both.

WORDS direct the content of a message

EMOTIONS accentuate and clarify their meaning.

Generally, non-verbal manifestations of communication are considered more reliable than its verbal counterparts in children. Children especially under the age of three are unable to properly verbalize their feelings through words and body language. However, this is more easily misunderstood than words because it can be interpreted in several ways. Assessment of nonverbal behaviour occurs in relation to the verbal content expressed, and the sender must validate the meaning of it. When communication is limited by a child's state of health, the field worker should pay even closer attention to nonverbal cues. Fear, anger, happiness and apathy can be assessed through facial expressions of the children.

Posture and gestures accompanying a verbal message are other forms of nonverbal behaviour associated with the overall process of communication.

COMMON SCENARIOS OF NON-VERBAL COMMUNICATION:
- *Lethargic and hopeless: a slumped, head-down posture and slow movements.*
- *Confidence and self-control: an erect posture and precise movements.*
- *Anxiety: rapid breathing diffuse, agitated body.*
- *Anger: movements that are more forceful and have less focus of direction.*

It is important to assess whether Nonverbal behaviour is an occasional occurrence, or is a generalized pattern of communication. A slumped posture in those who normally carry themselves well is a matter for greater concern, perhaps, than those in whom this is a persistent way of communication. Knowledge of the child's nonverbal pattern of communication becomes imperative in assessing the nature and meaning of changes in behaviour.

Domains of Communication

In face-to-face communication, a message is received through one or more of the five senses. In this way, a message originating in the external world is registered by the body and converted into internal experience. Messages are conveyed through the senses to the receiver primarily through the following domains:

Language

Composition of words which people use to share ideas and experiences with others.

Paralinguistic features

Features of a spoken message that are not contained in the words alone i.e. rhythm, pace, emphasis, intonation, pitch and tone of voice.

'I will see you at 8'o'clock' can be a simple declaration or a question, depending on the intonation. The tone of voice can be authoritative or persuasive.

These features help in the understanding and intervention of a message by giving the receiver evidence about the sender's state of mind.

In telephone conversations, paralinguistic features are particularly important because visual clues from the other person are missing.

Body language

These two words suggest that there is another channel for carrying meaning and communicating which does not use words at all. As every parent knows, a baby communicates effectively, if imprecisely, both

---

Non-verbal communication differs from verbal communication in that it is multi-channelled, deals with all senses, not just stimuli received through the sense of hearing.

The most important thing in communication is hearing what isn't being said.

-Anonymous

Accent and dialect can show social class and regional origins and differences.

BODY LANGUAGE
Communication via the movements or attitudes of the body

its urgent needs and satisfactions with gestures, non-verbal cries and noises. Each individual communicates through gestures and actions, or meaningful grunts and noises, to more articulated sounds, which eventually become the language. Visual signals also carry significant meaning and can replace, supplement or contradict a verbal message. Certain hand gestures, for example, are potent messages of affection or contempt, and exist across many cultures in different forms. While people are speaking, they gesture with their hands; some do it more than others do. They provide useful information as experiments have been shown in which people describe shapes or movements with or without using their hands.

Facial expressions

Possibly, because of their important survival value in infancy, subtle variations in smiles or looks are readily distinguished. Whether a child is pleased, puzzled or annoyed can be detected by observing the eyes and mouth.

Speech and gestures are controlled by the same area of the brain and develop in children simultaneously.

POSTURE
A characteristic way of positioning the body or its parts implicitly conveys a person's emotional or mental state.

Facial Expressions Associated with Different Emotions

	Eyes	Mouth	Face
Anguish/distress	Eyebrows down and together	Corners of lips turned down	Cheeks stretched
Anger/rage	Eyes narrow and alert	Lips curled under and tense	Facial muscles taut
Guilt/shame	Head down	May lick lips.	Some twitching of facial muscles
	Avoiding direct eye contact		
Happiness/joy	Life in the eyes	muscles relaxed	Face smiling
Contempt	Eyes narrowed and focused	Lips pursed	Jaws tense
		Tense with corners turned up	
Interest	Eyes wide open	Mouth open	Facial muscles relaxed
Fear	Eye contact limited	mouth closed	Muscles tense
Caring	Eyes soft	Smiling	Muscles relaxed

Eye contact

Eye contact is closely coordinated with speech: the speaker usually looks at the listener before making a major grammatical break and particularly before the end of utterances. Speakers often look away when they start to speak or are thinking about what they are saying. Cultural sensitivity regarding eye contact should always be kept in mind, as some cultures consider it an expression of confidence and truth, while others may consider it an expression of disobedience.

Body space and proximity

People need a certain space around them to feel comfortable, and this varies depending on age, sex and culture. Adults keep an arm's reach away from other people unless they know them reasonably well. When a field worker is physically handling children, this caution should be acknowledged.

Touch

This tells a good deal about the nature of a relationship, especially the degree of friendliness between two people. A gentle touch gives a message of care and affection by friends, relatives and children.

Physical Appearance

The manner and presentation of dress, hair, jewellery and make-up say a lot about an individual's personality, role, status and mood.

Field workers in their work settings may decide to wear proper and simple dress to build a good relationship with mother and child.

EFFECTIVE COMMUNICATION

Good Non-verbal Signals

Proximity:	Closer, lean forward if seated in front
Eye Contact:	More mutual gaze
Facial expression:	Smiling
Gestures:	Head nods, lively movements rather than arms on hips or folded.
Touch:	Gentle touch in an appropriate manner
Voice:	Higher pitch, upward contour, pure tone

EFFECTIVE COMMUNICATION

Good Non-verbal Practices

- *Do not gaze at the respondent for a longer time than is acceptable in the local culture: It is different for males and females.*
- *Avoid defensive and refusal postures which include postures such as the body being turned away from the speaker*
- *Use hand, finger and arm movements naturally; they should be neither too fast nor to slow.*
- *Listen attentively; direct attention to important points; create order in a confusing story by repeating the information in an organized form.*
- *Make physical touch according to culturally accepted norms.*

Communication Skills in Interviews

Effective communication plays a vital role in interviews (5) and it is a a prerequisite that the interviewer should be a good speaker as well as a good listener

Considerations for a good speaker

- Clarify your own concepts before communicating with the caregiver.
- Consider the human and physical setting
- Use a desirable and pleasant tone of voice and choice of language
- Speak clearly
- Repeat the key words or questions

L isten to what a person is saying, and not how he or she is saying it, as poor grammar, disorganized thought pattern and slow speech can make it difficult for the listener.

Considerations for a good listener

- Take time to listen and concentrate.
- Do not interrupt.

RESPONDING TO IMPOLITE OR HARSH (NON-COOPERATIVE) COMMUNICATION

- *Stay calm*
- *Stay polite*
- *Keep your tone of voice non-emotional*
- *Gently, ask for further clarification, if you have not understood the respondent*
- *Apologize if the respondent has understood wrongly*
- *Clarify your message*

Guidelines for Communication Skills with Respect to Interviewer

a) *Beginning the interview*

1. Greet the interviewee.

2. Introduce yourself and your organization.

3. Describe the purpose of the interview.

4. Expected amount of time for interview.

5. Take permission to document the information while interviewing.

b)   *The main part of the interview*

1. Maintain a positive atmosphere with warm manner and proper eye contact.

2. Listen carefully.

3. Be responsive to verbal and non-verbal cues.

4. Facilitate the interviewee, both verbally ('Tell me more') and non-verbally (using posture and head nods).

5. Encourage the interviewee to be relevant.

6. Show interest in caregiver and her child.

c)   *Ending the interview*

1. Ask if they would like to add anything.

2. Thank the respondent.

3. Take permission to leave / set next appointment.

Guidelines for Communication skills for various target groups in relation to ECD

1. Take some time to become familiar with child and parents.

2. Set up a physical environment that is warm, cheerful, and private and noise free.

3. If a child is becoming uncomfortable, question the parent how they usually help him to cope. Then use the same strategy as the parents use.

4. Do not go too close to the child until he / she becomes comfortable with you.

5. Observe the child's behaviour: if the child has maintained the eye contact, or starts asking questions, this shows that the child has become comfortable with your presence.

6. Encourage the child to ask questions during the interview with caregivers, as child may often feel ignored.

7. Use simple words for communication.

Communicating with Infants (0 to 18 months)

Infants in the early months communicate non-verbally e.g. smiling or crying. Young infants respond well to a calm physical touch. As the infant grows to about six months or more, stranger anxiety appears i.e. a child starts differentiating familiar and non-familiar faces. ECD workers need to make sure they are not talking directly to the child on the first visit. High pitched, soft voice and smile helps in building rapport.

Communicating with Toddlers (18 months to 3 years)

- These children have not yet fully developed verbal ability. As communication is mostly non-verbal, attention is required to pick non-verbal clues.

- Pushing the interviewer away with a frightened expression or crying is the sign of an uncomfortable child; if this happens, take help from the parents.

- Start talking to children by asking their names, and praising them. This helps them to understand that you are not there to harm them.

- Genuine praise fosters the communication process with this age group. Also, praise the child's belongings.

We are all inclined to judge ourselves by our ideals; others, by their acts.
-Harold Nicolson

- As their abstract thinking is still not developed, use simple words and short sentences, and repeat whatever you have said.

Communication with children (3 to 6 years)

- A child of this age group can express him/herself well through words. Initiate interaction with a child by having a conversation

  Where is he or she studying? /How many friends does he or she have?

- Let the child talk about anything he/she wants to, or let him/her sing a song. This will make the child comfortable with the assessor.

Communication with Caregivers

- Parents are the primary source of information about the child; keep a balance in your professional and friendly relationship.
- Keep taking the name of the child, as this will be a familiar means of expression for the parents.
- At times, the use of silence is helpful, especially when parents are talking about their child. Keep on nodding the head during the interview to express your concentration and attention.
- To some extent, do allow the parents to talk, even if it is beyond your objectives, particularly if they are sharing something about their child.

Counselling in the Context of ECD

Counselling is defined as the process by which the ECD worker (counsellor) helps caregivers clarify their issues related to childcare, and to decide upon further lines of action.

The Techniques

In ECD, two types of counselling have special importance for caregivers

a) Prescriptive Counselling

This refers to the counsellor's intention of recommending a particular solution or line of action.

> *After Kamal's finger was injured with a piece of glass while playing outside his home, Roshan suggested to the worried mother that she wash the injured surface with soap and water, wrap it with a clean bandage and take him immediately to the doctor for further care.*

b) Informative Counselling

This refers to the counsellor's intention to give additional information or education to the caregiver for situations related to childcare.

> *In the evening, Roshan again visited Kamal's house. After inquiring about Kamal's condition, she discussed with his mother the reasons and the importance of keeping the household surroundings clean and safe.*

Counselling Process

Conventionally, counselling has three stages (6)

Stage One:

> *If I am to speak ten minutes, I need a week for preparation; if fifteen minutes, three days; if half an hour, two days; if an hour, I am ready now.*
> -Woodrow Wilson

Problem Identification: Clarification of issues related to childcare practices

After the accident, Roshan had a thorough discussion with Kamal's mother as to why Kamal was injured. His mother placed all the blame on Kamal that he was a very naughty child, and it was very difficult to discipline him. Roshan pointed out family and community responsibilities to avoid such accidents with children.

Stage Two:
Goal setting: selection of preferred childcare practices

After detailed discussion, Kamal's mother concluded that there are several manageable and helpful ways to avoid unnecessary accidents among children, for example, there is lot of garbage in the surrounding area. When children play in unsupervised surroundings outside the home, without appropriate protective clothing, and without a proper play area, it is likely to lead to accidents.

Stage Three:
Action: moving towards the preferred child care practices

Both women decided to discuss these issues with caregivers living in the neighbourhood, and seek the help of community leaders to develop a safe play area for children in the community.

Counselling Skills
There are certain skills that are considered helpful in counselling (7) and can be learned and developed with practice. These are mainly categorized as verbal and non-verbal skills.

Non-Verbal Skills

a) Attention
It is the process of genuinely concentrating on the caregiver by being consciously aware of what the caregiver is trying to communicate or say. Reasonable eye contact and nodding are sympathetic touches, which are helpful in this regard.

b) Listening
Listening is the process of hearing and understanding the other person. It also helps listeners to note down the information

Verbal Skills

a) Questioning
Can be used primarily for first stage counselling, i.e. problem identification.

APPROPRIATE
* For problem exploration

"What happened? did Asghar develop diarrhoeal episodes?"

PROCESS OF COUNSELLING
* *Stage One: Problem Identification: Clarification of issues related to childcare practices*
* *Stage Two: Goal-setting: Selection of preferred childcare practices*
* *Stage Three: Action: Moving towards the preferred child care practices*

The most basic and powerful way to connect to another person is to listen. Just listen. Perhaps the most important thing we ever give each other is our attention.... A loving silence often has far more power to heal and to connect than the most well-intentioned words.
-Rachel Naomi Remen

- For further clarification

"Did you prepare ORS for him?"
"Do you mean your child has not eaten since then?"

INAPPROPRIATE
- Leading questions

"Did Kamal appear to be very sick?"

- Value-laden questions

"Did you make ORS for him with these dirty hands? "

- Confronting questions

"I have told you several times to prepare ORS properly, but you never listened to it carefully. Did you do it properly?"

b) Focusing
Refers to the use of statements to direct the conversation from general to specific topics, and it helps to focus the discussion.

"Can you please tell me exactly what Kamal ate the night before he developed diarrhoea?"

c) Reflection
The process of paraphrasing or repeating the last few words that the caregiver has used. The purpose is to encourage the caregiver to talk more explicitly and in detail about the topic under discussion.

"Yes, besides rice, what did he eat?"

d) Empathy
It refers to statements made by the ECD counsellor to the caregiver, so that she understands the situation and feelings of the caregiver.

"You must be quite upset and disturbed because your son is so ill"

e) Checking for understanding
Checking for understanding is important, to check whether the content of the conversational message is adequately understood and retained:
- By directly telling the caregiver that you have understood them completely.
- Indirectly, asking the caregiver to summarize the conversation for you.

"As we have just discussed, can you tell me what steps you will take in order to prevent such episodes of illness in future?"

IMPORTANT QUALITIES OF THE GOOD ECD COUNSELLOR

- *Show respect for the caregivers and children*
- *Do not judge them*
- *Do not overemphasize by using 'should' and 'ought' in communication*
- *Be Patient, do not expect the caregiver to follow your advice immediately*
- *Be Empathetic, listen to both what is said and what is implied*
- *Be Positive; do not blame the caregiver. The point is that a non-conducive situation for ECD has occurred, and the caregiver is trying to find ways of dealing with it*
- *Be willing to share yourself and your experiences with the caregiver if it seems to be helpful*
- *Do not automatically compare the caregiver's experience with your own experience*
- *Do not immediately comment on the caregiver's cultural values and perceptions*

Summary

- **Communication** means the sharing of thoughts, either in verbal or non-verbal fashion; it consists of sender, message, receiver and feedback.

- **Effective communication** requires skills and sensitivity from both sender and receiver.

- **Verbal communication** is dependent on words, while **nonverbal communication** is carried on through facial expression, body movements and gestures.

- **Domains of face-to-face communication** are dependent on the five senses and they receive information through language, paralinguistic features, body language, facial expressions, eye contact, body space and proximity, physical touch and physical appearance.

- **The Interviewer** requires skills of both a speaker and a listener for effective communication.

- **Counselling in the Context of ECD** is the process by which the ECD worker (counsellor) helps the caregiver clarify issues related to childcare, and to decide upon further lines of action.

- **Prescriptive Counselling** is primarily focused on advice for problem solving, while **Informative Counselling** is primarily focused on educating the caregiver regarding ECD.

- **Process of Counselling** comprises problem identification regarding the child, goal setting for the preferred action towards achieving better growth and developmental status of child.

- **Counselling Skills** can be developed with practice. Commonly required **Verbal Skills** are questioning, focusing, reflection, empathy and checking for understanding, while **Non Verbal Skills** are attention and listening.

There is only one pretty child in the world, and every mother has it.
-Chinese Proverb

The reason birds can fly and we can't is simply that they have perfect faith, for to have faith is to have wings **"**

-James Matthew Barrie

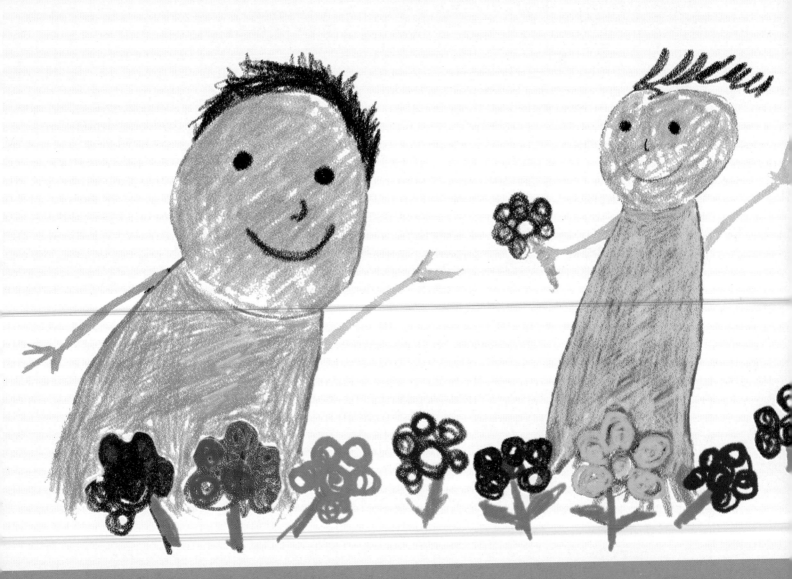

Artist:
Arfa
Age: 5 years

COMMUNITY-BASED PROGRAMMING

COMMUNITY

$\mathcal{D}$YNAMICS

*O*n an early October morning, while walking through a field, the sounds of roosters crowing and birds chirping are heard. Cattle are being herded by women towards grazing grounds. Men have already begun their work in fields and orchards – this appears to be a farm-based community.

We switch to another morning and another setting; here one can hear the roar of traffic, exhaust fumes fill the air, and crowds of people are moving quickly to begin work perhaps in a factory or a bank or an office building – this appears to be a non-farm-based community.

Community

The term community refers to a group, which has something in common. This generally means a common culture, language, common interests and identity, common set of values and beliefs (1). In terms of early childhood development, it is extremely important to understand the role of community i.e., composition and how it influences children. Communities vary across the world; they may be global, national, rural or urban communities. There is generally no upper limit to the number of people who belong to a community nor is one limited to being a member of just one community.

*A*person may belong to the Punjabi community, be part of the Pakistani community and be a member of the Muslim community – all at the same time.

COMMUNITY DYNAMICS
*Different communities
have different child rearing
practices and traditions,
and value knowledge and
skills in a manner which
differs for children and
adults.*

In addition, communities generally work together towards achieving a common set of goals (2). Working together requires a sufficiently organized social system to be able to achieve common goals, and to unite for common action. A shared culture facilitates organization, communication and joint action.

> **SOCIAL CLASS:** *relative economic and social positions within any given society (3).*
> * *A community usually has its own three broad groups*
>   * *upper socio-economic class*
>   * *middle socio-economic class*
>   * *lower socio-economic class (also called poverty level)*
> * *For individual families, the designation is based on the*
>   * *Income*
>   * *Occupation*
>   * *Area of residence and*
>   * *Education of the adults in the household*

Types of Community

Differentiating between farm based and non-farm-based communities is extremely important for the purpose of Early Childhood Development, as social and physical environments have important differences in terms of mediums for sensory stimulation of children.

In a *farm-based community (rural)* livelihood is generally linked to harvesting and cultivating available natural resources through farming, fishing, raising livestock, etc. It provides a contrasting environment in comparison to a *non-farm-based (urban)* environment, where the majority of the population is isolated from the farming culture, and where livelihood is linked more to the manufacturing and service oriented sectors, and families have greater access to manufactured products (4).

	Farm-based Communities (Rural)	Non-farm-based Communities (Urban)
Living Style	People generally live in separate housing structures. It is usually spread out and is less densely populated.	Size of the population is large, generally clustered and densely populated.
Income	Agriculture and livestock rearing is the main source of income. Most family members work in the fields.	Jobs related to industries are the main source of income.
Education	Comparatively low levels of literacy and less access to health facilities in terms of availability of transport and long distances to reach these facilities.	Higher overall levels of literacy and better access to facilities in terms of transport.
Tradition	Traditionally ascribed status plays an important part, as established by familial or tribal affiliations.	Economic resources and education standard may be considered more important.

Community Orientation

Learning about or having an orientation about a particular community is of primary importance in the implementation of developmental or research-related activities for early childhood development. It requires one's frequent interaction with members of the community, for developing better understanding about environmental and cultural aspects of the community (5). In addition, it also helps to understand about different vulnerable groups in the communities, such as pregnant women, old people and children as well as the community's power dynamics. Community assessment for ECD program activities usually refers to gathering general information on the following list of indicators:

1. Geographical boundaries of the community.
2. Demographics: race, ethnicity, gender ratio, age, economic standing, and educational level.
3. Cultural and religious value system.
4. Status of mother and child: physical, social, emotional and economic condition.
5. Sources of income.
6. Key people and leaders in the community.
7. Major concerns of the community in relation to child development.
8. Assurance and readiness for involvement in ECD program activities.
9. Potential partners and competitors.

Significance of Community Orientation

Learning about a community is important if:

1. One wants to work in partnership with a community, and for the intervention to be sustainable (to last even after the program team has left).
2. It increases understanding of the means to approach a community, and to tailor an intervention according to community needs.
3. The information collected can also be shared with others who want to work with the same community; it is used to measure change over the time spent working with the community. It can also be used to provide a profile of a community, in reports and proposals.

Selecting a Community for ECD Programs

There are some general considerations, which should be kept in mind when selecting an appropriate community for implementation of an early childhood development program:

Responsiveness: It is generally easier to work in a community where the leader is cooperative and is listened to by the community members. Some places are harder to penetrate than others, as in instances where getting permission from a community head might prove difficult, such as in cases where the community leader feels that the community's interests will not be served by external elements.

Motivation: It is important to meet with representatives of a community, to explore the need for planned developmental activities or intervention. It makes more sense to work in an area where the community members are enthusiastic for an ECD initiative in their communities.

Needs: Similarly, the community selected should be one in which you want to initiate your ECD endeavours, because in your opinion that community's ECD status requires improvement.

Accessibility: Initially work should be started on those communities, which are physically more accessible. Later, as resources permit, activities can be expanded to remote areas as well.

> *Our greatest natural resource is the minds of our children.*
> -Walt Disney

> *The old notion that children are the private property of parents dies very slowly. In reality, no parent raises a child alone.*
> -Marian Wright Edelman

Important queries that may help in community identification:

- *Where is the community located?*
- *How is the community organized? (Social class, ethnic groups, language spoken, and religion)*
- *Who are the community leaders?*
- *In your opinion what are the major problems of this community related to ECD?*
- *What is the community doing for the solution of these problems?*
- *Is there any other organization working in this community?*
- *Who is already doing something formally about ECD in the community? (NGOs, CBOs)*
- *What are they doing?*
- *How is it going?*
- *Which strategies are effective?*
- *Could we collaborate with them?*
- *Who else do we know who might be interested in this issue, such as health personnel, teachers, social mobilizers, religious and welfare organizations etc.(3)*

Abena was worried about the nutritional status of children in a nearby community. She first discussed the potential problem with the community leaders. After educating and sensitizing them about the issue, she asked them to identify and provide people from the community who could collaborate with her for the ECD cause. She was surprised to know that most of the community members were enthusiastic about supporting her cause.

> *There is no finer investment for any community than putting milk into babies.*
> *-Winston Churchill*

Summary

- **"Community"** refers to a group, which has something in common, and in terms of early childhood development, it is extremely important to understand the role of community, as it also serves as the social environment of a child.

- **Farm-based communities (rural)** are generally linked to harvesting and cultivating available natural resources through farming, fishing, raising livestock, etc.

- **Non-farm-based (urban)** environment where livelihood is linked more to the manufacturing and service-oriented sectors with greater access to manufactured products.

- **ECD communities** generally work together towards achieving a common set of goals, through a sufficiently organized social system. A shared culture facilitates organization, communication and joint action.

- **Orientation** of a particular community gives valuable information regarding existence of different vulnerable groups, and of the community's power dynamics, which is essential since ECD programmes are collaborative partnerships.

> *What's done to children, they will do to society.*
> *-Karl Menninger*

ECD PROGRAM

DEVELOPMENT

The clinic is crowded with people who have brought the sick to this facility. A middle-aged man walks into his room along with a woman and a 10-year-old child. The man wishes to show his sick son to the doctor. The parents complained that for the past one week he has been having episodes of diarrhoea and that his weight has reduced a lot. On examination, the doctor finds that the boy is malnourished. He appears to be small in height for his age and his daily diet in the afternoon included stuff from the thaylay walla (street vendor) outside his school. His parents complained that he skiped classes in school, and is beaten up by the schoolteacher for not doing his homework on time, and sleeping during lessons. There is no proper toilet facility available and the students have to go outside to relieve themselves near the garbage dump adjacent to the school.

For the doctor this is a common situation, and he knows that there are several children like this; deprived of the basic health and education amenities. Community based health and education facilities are being provided by different government as well as non-governmental service providers but they fall short of addressing these issues at an early age due to lack of collaboration, which in his view is important because of possible long-term implications on physical, socio emotional as well as cognitive function in later childhood. He is of the opinion that for these underprivileged rural children, an integrated early childhood development approach should be taken up at the community level.

What would be your approach in developing an integrated early childhood development program?

COMMUNITY-BASED ECD PROGRAM

Comprehensive provision of care in homes and communities to children from birth to six years of age, based on an integrated approach to

- *Augment nutrition, health and therapeutic service*
- *Promote sensory stimulation, developmental opportunities and education*
- *Encourage emotional support,*
- *Ensure safety and security,*
- *Improve water and sanitation quality*

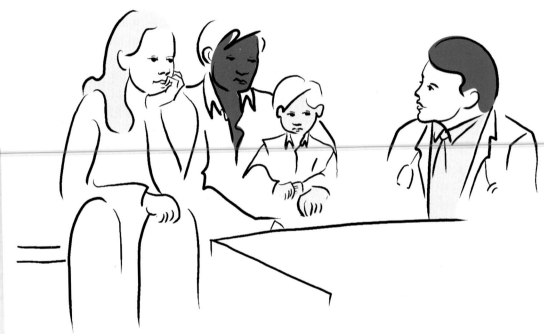

Community-based ECD program

The concept of intervening early in human life by providing adequate care and support is not a new idea. Biomedical research confirms (1) the importance of early childhood experiences in the development of the human brain. Scientific evidence also shows that most cognitive functions in later life are consequences of health, nutritional, educational and economic status early in life (2). ECD is crucial to human development and is a way to achieve community development. Strengthening quality of life of children, through improved nutrition, health and education, is a crucial part of community development and hence the development of nations. ECD programs can have positive long-term benefits including gains on future adult productivity (3). Underprivileged children reached by these programs would be able to enrol in schools, and can demonstrate better school performance through these programs (4, 5).

The success of an ECD program depends on its development as part of an organized strategy of outreach to susceptible communities. Therefore, a community based ECD program is crucial since it has the capacity to recognize different problems, and promote understanding of good caring practices at an early stage of child development. This is possible through outlining strategies that benefit not only children but also entire families involved in care giving. Since mothers are responsible for caring at the initial stages, the purpose of such a program is to allow caregivers to take an active role in the development of their children in several areas of caring, such as nutrition, access to schooling, and opportunities for play and sensory stimulation. A well-designed ECD program also offers community members the opportunities to develop individual skills enabling them to have better prospects of income generation (3).

ECD COMMUNITY DEVELOPMENTAL PROGRAMS
Create and support a network of individuals to assist in programs for Early Childhood Care in a community. This allows the community to take an active role in developing and advocating programs suited to their own needs, and providing a favourable environment for ECD. These programs can have components of research as well.

ECD RESEARCH PROGRAMS
Systematic and purposeful investigations for early childhood problems, to identify reasons relating to these problems. Conventional service provision is not included in ECD research programs.

Integration of program components at the level of children and their families, community leaders, education and health care providers in both public and private sectors ensures success of an ECD program by addressing major aspects of care from conception to early years of schooling. Furthermore, sustainability of ECD programs is possible when there is suitable coordination and interaction between the different stakeholders.

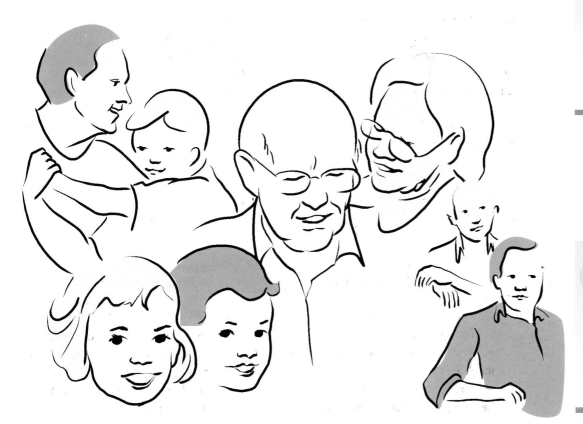

EARLY CHILDHOOD DEVELOPMENT PRACTITIONER
It is a sub-group of caregivers, who are professionally capable and responsible for providing services related to care and nurturance during early childhood.

SUSTAINABILITY
Capability of an ECD program ensuring continuity of its initiatives for an extended period through efficient use of resources, commitment and provision of services by involving the community

"In the end, poverty, putridity and pestilence; work, wealth and worry; health, happiness and hell, all simmer down into village problems.
-Martin H. Fischer"

Planning Cycle for an ECD Program

Planning cycle is a systematic process of purposeful activities undertaken within given resources and time span (6). It is a methodical plan that identifies and clarifies ECD needs, selects the best way to meet the identified needs, implements the methods and evaluates the extent to which those needs are met for the plan of action.

ECD programs can consist of five basic stages as shown in Fig 1 below. We will discuss the stages in the following text.

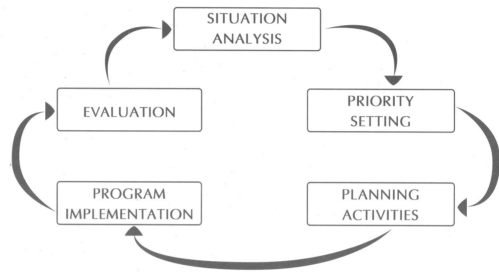

> *Without leaps of imagination, or dreaming, we lose the excitement of possibilities. Dreaming, after all, is a form of planning.*
> -Gloria Steinem

Information on the community's knowledge and attitude towards early childhood development is essential for planning an ECD program.

Situation Analysis

The first step of the planning cycle involves assessing the ECD needs of a community. These can be assessed through situation analysis, by evaluating the present situation from the perspective of parents, education and health care service providers, and the community as a whole. It is also possible to collect information regarding awareness and motivation level of community members in the context of ECD through situation analysis. This is accomplished by actual participation of community members in this process.

Situation analysis is important for understanding the infrastructure and resources of a community. Information on physical, social and cultural boundaries is crucial for becoming familiar with the community and sensitizing the community to the ECD programme (7).

Steps of Situation Analysis

The following aspects need to be considered during planning of situation analysis:

a) Where and how this information will be collected

A community setting should be identified where problems related to ECD are prevalent. This information can be obtained either from public or private sector organizations doing similar work. Participation of community members is extremely important for a planned collection of information at this stage. This can be done by involving the primary caregivers, health care providers, school staff, religious and community leaders in focus group discussions. Involvement of these groups may have an influence on situation analysis, hence care should be taken while selecting people for information gathering by including those individuals who have either some prior experience or necessary skills of conducting such activities. Baseline quantitative surveys on the same groups of people also give relevant ECD indicator information.

While developing ECD programs, the overall situation in the community that affects children's lives must be taken into account. This is because the programs that are developed can be affected by the existing state of social environment.

Information should be collected according to the goals of an ECD program. More specifically, it is essential to know what aspects of the community's needs can be covered through an ECD program. This information is organized in five categories of the social environment with respective examples, affecting child development (8, 9, 10).

- ### Internal relationships: child's interaction with family
  Information is collected on child's interaction with family such as parents, siblings and grand parents. This interaction should be determined to understand the nature of their immediate environment.
  - Child rearing practices
  - Opportunities for sensory stimulation

- ### External relationships: interaction in neighbourhood, school and playground
  Information of children's external relationships at the level of neighbourhood, school and immediate surroundings is important, since these interactions have a lifelong influence on their development.
  - Playing in the playground
  - Number of visits to other households in a week
  - Involvement of child in school activities such as drawing, telling stories and poems etc

- ### External services: Work place and community health services
  Information on parents' social setup, working conditions, and health and education facilities in the community creates a social and economic safety net, and opportunities for enhancement of growth and development.
  - Health infrastructure
  - Schooling facilities
  - Paid maternity and sick leave
  - Family health benefits offered by employer organization

- ### Socio-cultural and political context
  It is also imperative that information be obtained about national policies and government laws designed to ensure equitable opportunities in terms of health, nutrition, and education for child development. Information on the community's culture and customs also gives an insight into practices that are related to child development.
  - Joint family system
  - Primary schools for girls
  - Gender preference in utilization of health care services

- ### Significant life events
  Information about major life events is also important since this brings changes in child's existing relationships and influences its development.
  - Sibling's birth
  - Admission in school
  - Moving to a new neighbourhood

We all live with the objective of being happy; our lives are all different and yet the same.
-Anne Frank

ECD RELATED SOCIAL SERVICES
- **Health care**
  - *Dispensaries, hospitals*
  - *Doctors*
  - *Paramedical staff*
  - *Medicines*
- **Education**
  - *Schools*
  - *Trained teachers*
- **Public works**
  - *Piped water*
  - *Sewage system*
  - *Electricity and natural gas*
  - *Play area*
- **Social welfare setup**
  - *Free ambulance service*
  - *Shelter for the homeless*

b) Collaboration with caregivers for an ECD program

Collaboration with caregivers is important since they provide psychological and emotional support to the child. An ECD program can undertake collaborative efforts with primary care givers such as parents, siblings and grandparents as well as with social service providers to obtain information that can be used to structure and further organize an ECD program for children as well as caregivers.

c) Needs Assessment

One of the purposes of carrying out situation analysis is to collect the information needed specifically for program design, and identifying sources to seek this information (11). This can be done directly by asking individuals in the community or by observing their behaviour.

ECD needs assessment of a particular community should be in consultation with the community itself, as it helps in reaching agreement. It also ensures community support for your program. Information on ECD needs can be acquired for different categories, through different sources.

Information on the geography and physical infrastructure of the community is where needs assessment should begin. Information should be collected on demography, socio-economic and political situation, community organizations and resources. Information can also be collected that is specifically related to ECD indicators such as access to health and education facilities, nutrition, economic conditions, social interaction, sensory stimulation and play.

i. Sources

There are three primary methods of collecting information on the needs of a community. These are visits, baseline surveys and the study of existing documents.

1) *Visits (Observations):* are sometimes considered the most direct method of collecting needs assessment data, although in many cases, a great deal is involved in interpreting observations.
   - Observe water supply of a household: piped water or well water
   - Observe sewage disposal: through open or covered lines

2) *Baseline Surveys (Interviews):* are considered the easiest way of collecting needs assessment data. Questionnaire-based interviews and focus groups discussions are also effective methods of gathering information. However, what people tell and actually do may differ. It is sometimes important to verify the results of interviews with observations and document analysis.

3) *Documentation Review:* e.g., looking at birth, health facility or school records can provide useful needs assessment data. However, in some situations, it may be difficult or impossible to obtain the desired documents.

ii. ECD Indicators

Community based ECD programs can address nutrition and care-related developmental issues through observations of children's physical growth, social behaviour and language, by the assessment of nutrition, health, education and developmental indicators in the community setting. Indicators help define the geographic, socio-economic or ethnic groups most in need of attention.

ECD REINFORCEMENTS
Comprehensively collected information reflects the needs for respective community based ECD programs.

"If you have built castles in the air, your work need not be lost; that is where they should be. Now put the foundations under them."
-Henry David Thoreau

"One may miss the mark by aiming too high as too low."
-Thomas Fuller

Table 1: Common ECD Indicators with respect to social environment model *

Internal relationships: child's interaction with family	
Child rearing practices	Availability of balanced diet
	Quality time given by parents to children
Sensory stimulation	Learning material provided to the child
Safe physical environment	Covered rotary fan
	Protected stairs
	Medicines kept out of reach of children
	Sharp, pointed tools kept out of reach of children
External relationships: interaction in neighbourhood, school and playgrounds	
Gross motor	Running and jumping (refers to large muscle movements)
Fine motor	Drawing pictures or stacking small blocks (refers to small muscle movements and control)
Cognitive development	Ask questions about events and objects (curiosity)
	Sorting blocks of different colours (differentiation)
	Work with puzzles (problem solving)
Emotional development	Child is happy on seeing parents, siblings (expression and comprehension of emotion)
Social development	Interaction with family and peers (socialization skills)
Language comprehension	Understanding of verbal communication
Language production	Verbal communication of thought
External services: work place and community health services	
Immunization status	Coverage of children according to 6 recommended childhood vaccines
Maternal Health care	Antenatal care received through trained health professionals
Community level facilities	Structure of health facilities: doctors, nurses and dispensaries available
	Schools in the community and up to what level
	Piped water or through tankers, wells
	Playgrounds in the community
	Covered sewage lines in the community
Child growth and developmental status	
Anthropometric assessments	Based on height or weight for age, height for weight
Low birth weight (LBW)	Children weighing less than 2500 grams at birth
Infant mortality rate (IMR)	Deaths per 1000 live births among infants
Child mortality (under five)	Deaths per 1000 live births among children aged under 5 years
Socio cultural and political context	
National policy	Primary schools for girls
	Implementation of child labour laws in the community
Culture & customs	Joint or nuclear family system
Significant life events	
Educational	Admission to a school
	Children repeating classes
	Drop-out from schools
Family	Death of immediate family member, e.g. father, mother, grandparents or siblings
	Birth of siblings
	Marriage of surviving parent

* Details of social environment are given in Chapter 2

d) Organization of information and analysis

Finally, once information on needs of the community regarding ECD has been collected, it can be presented in tabulated forms for a quick review. Information must be carefully synthesized for proper understanding and communication.

Priority Setting

ECD programs based on evidence and context are able to prioritize a child's needs for optimal growth and development for the respective community. This also gives the opportunity of prioritizing the program according to existing facilities in the community in terms of material, human and educational resources (12).

ECD programs are built on the strengths of the community, such as a strong desire of the parents to provide better opportunities in life to their children. Many problems may be present in the community or area. No one organization or group can solve all these problems. They address only those, which match their resources, interests and goals.

a) Priority setting: a collaborative exercise

Community participation can increase the effectiveness of an ECD program during the implementation phase; therefore, communities are involved in establishing priorities by building local capacity to identify needs and then seek solutions. It gives them a sense of ownership and they can be held accountable at later stages. Collective participation encourages unity and strength within the community and is important to ensure that decisions taken will be implemented and programs maintained once initial support is withdrawn.

> **ECD PROGRAMMING PRIORITY SETTING PRINCIPLES**
> *Child centred Community development*
> - *A child's development is influenced by its environment, includes home, community, institution and culture.*
>
> *Integration of childcare and social services*
> - *An ECD program should be able to function across different levels of the community, starting with the child, and including caregivers, community leaders, schools, teachers, doctors and other organizations working in the area.*

b) Community Participation in ECD program development

Community members are the main stakeholders in any ECD program. From this perspective, the aim of the program should be to increase community participation at initial stages of situation analysis and ECD program development, to obtain their constructive input on program design, goals and objectives. Their involvement ensures that an ECD program is:

- Efficient: community members provide a broader knowledge base
- Effective: community views are incorporated in design
- Sustainable: community is encouraged to take initiatives based on their knowledge, and acquire   skills to maintain benefits once the program ends

Community participation formally begins with formation of a community based ECD committee. Its members can be people from the ECD program team and representative leaders of the area where the program is to be started. People from other segments such as direct caregivers (parents), people with similar prior experience, religious leaders, and those service providers working in either public or private sectors can be included in this community ECD committee.

Investing in preventive programs is more cost-effective as compared to compensatory programs.

Map out your future, but do it in pencil.
-Jon Bon Jovi

c) Perspective of Community Leaders and other stakeholders

Once a community ECD committee has been formed it provides a forum to members of the community to express their concerns and views on issues related to ECD in their setting. Communication is vital since it creates a setting for all the concerned people of the community, and for establishing a relationship of trust, and for discussing mutual concerns, and previous experiences with each other. Focus group discussions can be held to ascertain views of different segments of the community.

d) Life cycle approach

Life cycle approach for holistic human development is vital in priority settings for ECD programming. ECD does not start from the child, rather it begins from the mother whose physical and mental health even prior to conception has a direct influence on later foetal development and childbirth. Low birth weight babies are more likely to have a childhood of impaired development and poor physical health, giving rise to stunted adolescents with compromised physical and mental capabilities. Consequently as adults, they have reduced capacity to produce healthy babies and provide care to them. They are at increased risk of having, babies with intrauterine growth retardation (IUGR), stillbirths, miscarriages and foetuses with impaired brain development. This creates a vicious circle that needs to be broken (13). A sound situation analysis will give relevant information about on what stage an intervention is required in a particular community.

> *What cannot be achieved in one lifetime will happen when one lifetime is joined to another.*
> *-Harold Kushner*

e) Setting Objectives

Objectives are defined as statements that express the intended results of the activities of a program (14). While setting up objectives we need to consider the following points:

Characteristic	Description	Example	Reasoning
Explicit	Objectives should be precise and clear	To provide primary health care facilities to all children aged up to 5 years by 2010	Explicitly giving the target age group and duration of the program
Quantifiable	Objective should be measurable at the end of the program	To estimate the number of children who were born with Low Birth Weight (LBW)	Both number and weight of the children can be "measured"
Realistic	Objectives should be achievable	To provide tetanus toxoid vaccines at the village medical facility	Provision of vaccines at a particular village medical facility is achievable
Applicable	Objectives are related to the specific needs	To improve the community's water supply by repairing the leakages through water pipes	It is applicable if in the scope of the community
Time-Bound	Objectives are achievable within a given time frame	To immunize pregnant mothers with tetanus toxoid in a district	It can be achieved by following a timetable of 1 year

f) Identification of Problems and Challenges

During designing of a program, issues of central importance should be identified to ensure that the program contributes to the maximum benefit of children in the community e.g., while designing a program to reduce malnutrition among children, start by identifying the age group most commonly affected, and the type of the diet available to them. However, the parents might insist that they need the doctor from the program to treat their children, rather than to receive education and bring improvement in their diet. It might also be discovered that children of a particular ethnic group are affected more than children in other groups, and the program may want to invest more on that high-risk group resulting in the program being blamed

ECD REINFORCEMENTS
Income generation
ECD programs should encourage income generation prospects of caregivers through capacity building initiatives for individual members of the community, enabling program sustenance without external help.

The challenge for the program team is to suggest a method, which takes into account the power relations among groups of caregivers responsible for program objectives.

for not assisting all the groups equally. If benefiting a particular group is likely to be the effect of a potential ECD program, then this needs to be brought to the attention of all the participants.

Another challenge for ECD programs is creating employment opportunities for primary caregivers as this has an effect on the social environment of the child.

ECD REINFORCEMENTS
Caregiver employment
Mother's employment effects on children are positive in general, particularly for girls, by creating:
- *Confident maternal image*
- *More provision of resources*
- *Increased decision power*
- *Modified allocation of labour*

STRATEGY
Choosing a method and carrying it out to meet the set objectives
PLANNING
Developing a work plan for implementation of strategies to achieve ECD objectives within a given period

Planning activities

Once problems are identified and objectives set, appropriate strategies need to be developed. When a problem has been identified (needs assessment) and a priority set with a decision on what has to be achieved (setting objectives), the next step is to plan activities according to the list of the objectives. The community ECD committee can then come up with the ways and means by which the set objectives are to be achieved. These ways and means are also known as strategies (14).

In planning, strategy means a statement that describes the broad approach to achieve an objective. Early childhood development is not possible by adopting a single strategy. This is because the overall environment, including peers, caregivers, teachers, health services personnel, and religion affect the development of children and community leaders, play areas, marketplace etc. Hence, a mix of strategies is needed with a multidisciplinary approach by involving different segments of the community. Since the choice of strategies is dependent upon the objectives that are to be achieved, some of the strategies that can be adopted are:

Strategy 1:	**Delivery of child health care services**
Objective:	*To improve vaccination status of children*
Target group:	*children < 5 years old*
Approach:	*Provision of vaccines to the available community based facilities*

(The immediate aim of this strategy is to make an improvement in the child's overall development. Childhood vaccination is one example. Other objectives can be promoting nutrition, improving survival, preparing the child for school, improving child socialization. These services can be provided at home, through medical facilities, community centre or a local meeting place. These services can also be provided through newspapers, radio or television).

Strategy 2:	**Education of caregivers**
Objective:	*To change caregivers' attitude regarding prelacteal feed to the newborn*

Target group:	*Grandmothers, pregnant mothers and mothers of young children.*
Approach:	*Education courses for mothers*

(The broad objective for this strategy is to create awareness about the importance of the caregiver's role with regard to child's development and to change harmful practices and customs such as physical punishment or gender biases for the child's as well as mother's benefit. Care should be taken while providing information, which should be culturally appropriate)

Strategy 3:	**Promotion of community development**
Objective:	*Mobilizing community to meet the health needs of pregnant women*
Target group:	*Community members*
Approach:	*Social mobilization: conduct meetings with community members to determine their needs and priorities.*

(This can provide a base for the community to take action on its own, sensitize them to the mother's needs and participate in programs providing services to mothers and children living in their locality)

Strategy 4:	**Increase demand for ECD initiatives**
Objective:	*To increase demand for better opportunities for children regarding education, health and social aspects by the community members and caregivers*
Target group:	*Community members and caregivers*
Approach:	*To create awareness of the benefits of having better development opportunities for children in the context of the larger interest of the community or country*

> *For every complex problem there is a simple solution that is wrong.*
> -George Bernard Shaw

PROGRAMMING STRATEGIES PRINCIPLES

Delivery of quality childcare services

Delivery of childcare services targeting health, nutrition, sensory stimulation and education aspects of early childhood should account for the timeliness, cost-effectiveness and sustainability of services.

Practical education of caregivers

Education sessions for parents should focus on what to expect from children in different age groups and how to respond to their specific needs.

Promotion of integrated community development

ECD programmes ensure availability of optimal resources for children without any duplication. This is done by collective participation of caregivers, community members and education, health and other social service providers.

Increase demand for ECD initiatives

ECD programmes increase the level of awareness and motivation of caregivers and community members regarding the importance of ECD initiatives, thereby increasing the demand for such initiatives; and consequentially driving the supply from concerned entities.

Program Protocol Documentation

One of the important steps after developing a program framework is to develop a protocol that should act as a blueprint for implementation of the program (15). It is a process of writing down all the steps mentioned above in a systematic manners as one document.

Following are the components of protocol development:

a) Program summary

The purpose of writing a summary for the program is to present the salient features of the program in a few sentences, so that they can have a brief overview of the program without going into details. The summary usually includes the background or status of problems that are encountered in the community regarding ECD objectives, program design and the programmed benefits to the target group or community through this program.

b) Problem Statement

This statement is needed to convince the community that the program is extremely important and is much needed. Background information about the community affected is collected and is recorded in this statement. References are made for the reports that have already been done, with some groundwork on the problem to support the statement of the community workers.

c) Statement of Objectives

An objective is the statement of what result is to be achieved after a certain period. In general, more than one objective is needed to achieve the desired results. The objectives provide the guidelines for developing a methodology for the programme, and help convert ideas into actions.

d) ECD Program Design

This step of protocol development is where decision is made on achievement of objectives. The design of the program will emerge once decision about premises for the activity, services that are to be provided through the programme, the delivery system, work force needed, and the training are provided.

e) Budget

Once the above steps of protocol development are completed, a financial plan to operate the program is needed. In order to have long-term sustainability of the program, it is important to make a budget by utilizing the local resources that are available. To facilitate this process, a list of expected expenses for the different components is made. These components can include basic salaries and allowances, cost of equipment and supplies, cost of utility bills, stationery and miscellaneous costs for unforeseen expenses.

> *Shoot for the moon. Even if you miss, you'll land among the stars.*
> *-Les Brown*

> **ECD PROGRAM DESIGN**
> *It is an organized framework of specific information giving details of selected community based strategies and period of program implementation.*

Summary

- **Community based ECD programs** are crucial for human development and for achievement of community development. Strengthening quality of life of children, through improved nutrition, health and education, is a vital part of a community based ECD development programme.

- **Planning the cycle for an ECD program** is a systematic process of purposeful activities undertaken within given resources and time span. It is a methodical plan comprising various stages, which are situation analysis, priority setting, planning activities, program implementation and evaluation.

- **Situation analysis** involves assessing the ECD needs of a community. Collected information covers perspectives of parents, education and health care service providers, and the community as a whole. Through participation of community members in this process, awareness and motivation level of community members in the context of ECD is also assessed. Three main sources of information are *visits, baseline surveys and documentation reviews.*

- **Priority setting** in ECD programs is based on evidence. It thus prioritizes child needs for optimal growth and development for the respective community. ECD programs are prioritized according to what already exists in the community in terms of material, human and educational resources.

- **Objectives** of an ECD program should be explicit, quantifiable, realistic, applicable and achievable within a given timeframe.

- **Strategies** for an ECD program are developed once problems are identified and objectives set. Diverse strategies are needed for ECD programs, with a multidisciplinary approach by involving different segments of the community.

- **Program protocol documentation** is a process of writing the program summary, problem statement, objectives, program design and budget to act as a blueprint for ECD program implementation.

> *The best time to plant a tree is twenty years ago. The second best time is now.*
>
> *-African Proverb*

ECD PROGRAM

MANAGEMENT

Maria had been given the responsibility of implementing an ECD program for mothers and their children in Sanwal village. The program focused on application of new strategies for child development, and was to be done in collaboration with local administrative staff, health care providers and private organizational setups. She had to start the program in two weeks time, and had a lot of work ahead in the days to come. Maria was quite pleased with the fact that she had just recently received training regarding ECD program implementation steps and strategies under a capacity-building program. She thought that now she would be able to do a good job.

> *We will either find a way, or make one.*
> *-Hannibal*

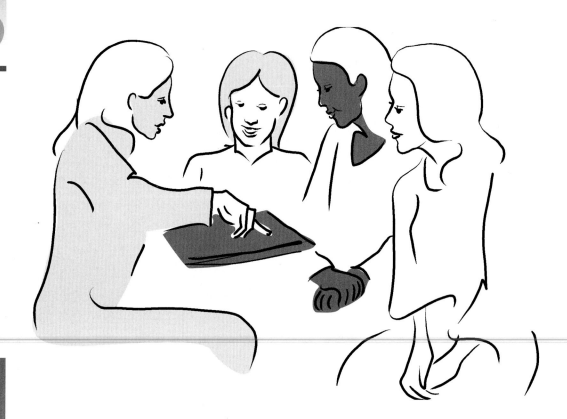

ECD PROGRAMS

Community based ECD Programs stem from the conventional thinking of education discipline, and aim at providing cognitive enrichment to preschoolers (aged 3 to 6) growing up in impoverished circumstances.
This may be too little, too late, in the perspective of brain development. In this context cognitive enrichment programs for infants (aged 0 to 3) would be more valuable and make better sense.

ECD program management covers overall planning and coordination of a program from inception to completion, is aimed at achieving program goals and ensuring completion on time, within cost and to the required quality standards (1).

Once an ECD program has been planned its implementation can be accomplished in various phases, beginning with identification of a community, formation of a community ECD committee, selection of a field ECD team, conducting baseline surveys and implementation of ECD activities in the community. A system of monitoring and evaluation is in place for quality check and quality assurance. Regular status reports are made through use of various measurement tools tracking program tasks. A designated person from the program staff (field coordinator) can carry out ECD Program implementation.

Program management is a skilful job and requires coordination at different levels (2). It is a multidisciplinary activity involving caregivers, schoolteachers, health care service providers, religious and community leaders. While building a team to implement ECD programs, all relevant sectors should be included. It is also necessary for this team to be capable of interacting with any other new sectors that need to be involved in community development activities within a particular setting.

ECD PROGRAM IMPLEMENTATION PHASES

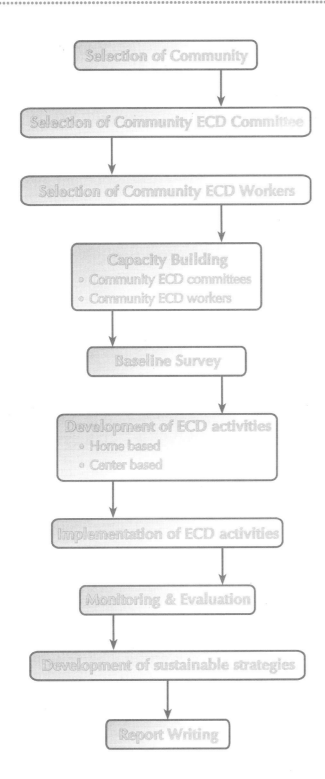

ECD PROJECTS
ECD projects are a planned course of action with specific work plans to achieve objectives.

I am a part of all that I have met.
-Alfred Tennyson

We have already discussed some general considerations for selection of communities for implementation of ECD programs in chapter 10. Here we will discuss some aspects of community participation and mobilization along with processes involved in selection of community leaders.

Community Participation in ECD Program Management

In the context of this book the term community participation refers to people participating in joint situation analysis and ECD program planning, which leads to action plans that can be transformed into a sustainable positive change in the ECD status of a community. The objective of using a participatory approach is to enable the community to take control over local decisions, to have a sense of ownership and a higher level of investment in any program or intervention strategy (3, 4).

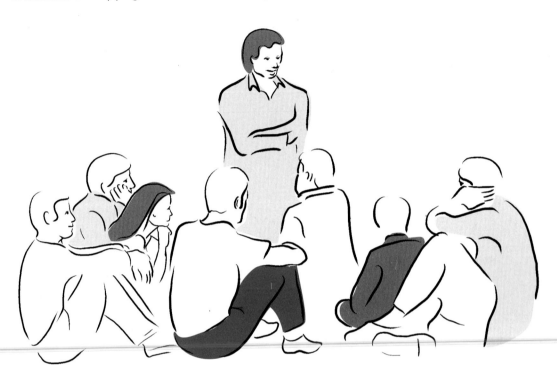

> *The sea rises, the light fails, lovers cling to each other, and children cling to us. The moment we cease to hold each other, the sea engulfs us and the light goes out.*
> -James Baldwin

LEADERSHIP
The capacity to influence the ideology and actions of the community, through the process of persuasion, towards achievement of a common goal

> *Inside my empty bottle I was constructing a lighthouse while all the others were making ships.*
> -Charles Simic

Community Mobilization in ECD Program Management

Community mobilization is a process through which people in a given community can be given common goals with the purpose of enabling them to work together, without prejudice to other members of the group (5). For ECD, community mobilization takes on the shape of a community movement where the care givers i.e. parents, siblings and other relatives interact with the health care providers, local political and religious leaders, teachers imparting education at schools along with the ECD program field team and other stakeholders. Community mobilization also starts a process of communication among ECD program stakeholders, assisting them in determining who, what, and how issues are decided. This interaction and extended communication facilitates a motivated and participatory decision-making process (6).

Community Leaders

Community leaders (also known as 'gatekeepers') are individuals or a group within a community whose support is essential for any community intervention. The role they play could be inherited or acquired depending on each individual case, and they generally are centres of power within communities (7).

Hence before beginning work in a community, it is extremely important to first contact community leaders and explain to them what you would like to do in the community, and get their support. For this, it is important to first identify community leaders.

Identification

Various strategies need to be applied in identifying community leaders depending on the circumstances; however, it is important to state that one should use one's best judgment. Strategies include:

- Contacting the local government representative.
- Contacting relevant public and private facilities located in close proximity to the community such as schools and Basic Health Units (BHUs).
- Identify possible NGOs or CBOs currently or previously functioning in the area for information.
- Within the community, a mosque may prove a good place to start as it is an openly approachable space and the Cleric is usually a community leader as well.
- The house of a respected community member or an open space can also be considered as a meeting place, where even the female community leaders can gather and participate.

Characteristics

Community leaders can be from any occupation, but they should have these characteristics:
- Members of the same community.
- Respected by other community members.
- Having a strong relationship with the community members.
- Able to persuade people in the community.
- In a position to give time to the community.

Once the processes of community identification, participation, mobilization and identification of leaders are complete, we go to the next phase of ECD program implementation, i.e. selection of the community ECD committee. However, before doing that we need to identify personnel who are responsible for this task, and in the case of ECD program management, this responsibility usually lies with the field coordinator.

Field Coordinator in an ECD Program

This position is responsible for coordination of the ongoing development and implementation process of an ECD program. Field coordinators work directly with community members, public and private sector service providers, educational institutions and other ancilliatory agencies to facilitate joint planning and decision-making to meet community needs. A field coordinator can provide direction and management oversight for different aspects of the program. Field coordinators also perform special assignments as and when required.

Responsibilities

The Field Coordinator should be involved in the ECD field team selection along with the community ECD committee. He / she should:

- Develop protocols for field activities in consultation with the community ECD committee.
- Organize training sessions for the ECD field team with respect to program requirements. The Field Coordinator should be well acquainted with the training material herself/himself, as the team should feel comfortable that whenever they have difficulty in understanding they can turn to this person for guidance regarding the task in hand.

When Jesus Christ asked little children to come to him, he didn't say only rich children, or White children, or children with two-parent families, or children who didn't have a mental or physical handicap. He said, "Let all children come unto me."
-Marian Wright Edelman

Important characteristics of a community leader
- *Respectful*
- *Dependable*
- *Persuasive*

QUALITY CHECK
Can be implemented by:
- Observing the performance of individual team members and making decisions on their further involvement in the program
- Conducting regular meetings for quality appraisal

- Coordinate with the community ECD committee and keep them informed of the status of the program in the community.
- Be responsible for financial management of the ECD program, with proper record keeping as in a logbook.
- Maintain the logistical requirements of the ECD program such as supplies of office equipment, stationery and transport etc.
- Laying down the Terms of Reference for the functioning of the community ECD committee and the ECD field team.
- Be responsible for resolution of conflicts that arise among the working members of a field ECD team.
- Implement Quality Check (QC) mechanisms.
- Report on the status of the ECD program to higher authorities.

ECD LEADERSHIP
Providing vision and guidance to the community for achieving ECD initiatives

She/he should have good leadership qualities and managerial skills as well as the ability to supervise a team of individuals working to achieve specific objectives within stipulated timeframes.

LEADERSHIP QUALITIES OF A FIELD COORDINATOR
- *Provides vision*
- *Aware of local perspectives of the community*
- *Good communicator (efficiently communities with all team members)*
- *Inspires confidence*
- *Mobilizes team members*
- *Accepts ownership for team decisions*
- *Knows how to encourage ECD team members*

MANAGERIAL QUALITIES OF A FIELD COORDINATOR
- *Uses available resources optimally*
- *Well versed in proper methods of selection, training and motivation*
- *Confident in decision making*
- *Gives the team members all the information they need to do their jobs*
- *Creates an atmosphere of growth*
- *Sets high standards*
- *Sets guidelines for team members' interaction with each other*

ECD MANAGER
Capacity to plan, organize, and direct resources for the community, through the process of administration and supervision, towards achievement of common ECD goals.

Note: In ECD programs that have a larger scope and involve a greater number of people working in a team, another post of a field supervisor can be created. A field supervisor can function as field related operations support person under the Field Coordinator. In these instances, steps must be taken to ensure proper maintenance of hierarchy.

Community ECD Committee

A committee can be formed of individuals from the program team and from the community. When selecting people from the community it is important to consider identification of "representative" community leaders and some "elders", who could be instrumental in getting your message across to the people of the area you are working in. Once a committee has been formed, it is very important to introduce the whole team to the selected group of people. This is possible by arranging a meeting with the newly formed committee and the members of your program team. This is so that everyone will know persons who are working in each context. It would then be possible for individual team members to develop working relationships with community leaders.

We were born to unite with our fellow men, and to join in community with the human race.
—Cicero

To start the process of forming a community ECD team, Maria contacted community leaders and informed them that she had come to their community to suggest implementation of an ECD program. She also explained to them that there was a need to form a community ECD team. This was necessary to facilitate community involvement and development through the program. Maria was glad to get the support of the community leaders, especially as they were very interested in the work she was doing, and because she was able to form a well represented community ECD committee due to proper announcement in the area.

The community can participate in the program in various ways, such as providing required space, furniture and most importantly human resources. While building associations within the community it is important to establish feelings of familiarity and confidence amongst community members and ECD program staff who are not from within the community.

Criteria for community ECD committee formation
- **Include people from different segments to have a wider representation of the community**
- **Include people with relevant experience and skills**
- **Select motivated individuals**

Terms of Reference for Community ECD Committee Formation

Once the community ECD committee has been formed, the Terms of Reference (TOR) should be laid down in consultation with the selected committee members. This is an important step in the formation of a community ECD committee, as it is meant to facilitate the future functioning of the program in participation with the community ECD committee. TOR acts as a protective document for all stakeholders involved in ECD program implementation.

GUIDELINES FOR TOR	
Objective	State the objective of the ECD program clearly for everyone to understand
Stakeholders	Those who can be affected by the objectives of the program
Representatives	Mention criteria for inclusion in the community ECD committee to ensure adequate representation in the community ECD committee from different segments of the community where the program is to be launched
Responsibilities	Assign responsibilities to members of the community ECD committee; this is important to gain comprehensive community participation
Discipline	Lay down guidelines for course of action in cases of misconduct on part of ECD program team members, community ECD committee members and ECD field team members
Meeting schedule	Set weekly/monthly meeting schedules with the community ECD committee to exchange information regarding the program and the community (such as response of community members to the program)
Venue	Location where the scheduled meetings can be held.
Timeframe of program	Provide the approximate time or duration for which the program is expected to last.
Quorum	A baseline quorum (e.g. 50%) for conducting community ECD committee meetings is necessary, especially for important policy decisions. A quorum is necessary to give validity to the decisions made during a meeting.

We're still not where we're going, but we're not where we were.
-Natash Jasefowitz

ECD Field Team Selection

Team selection comprises some "essential elements" that need to be considered when selecting or forming teams for a given task. As in other activities, program team selection also requires prior planning. The first step is to list the number and categories of positions to be filled.

If the number of interviewees is quite large, divide them into groups and assign different days and time slots to specific groups. Assign the responsibility to the relevant person about informing the candidates concerning date, time and venue to be given to the them. A checklist of the candidates is helpful in order to confirm whether all have been contacted or not.

Prepare points on the information required from the candidates, as well as the information you wish to give about your program, especially salary packages. That would help the interview in being more focused, and enable an objective assessment of the candidates.

Select the most appropriate person for the job, keeping in view the qualifications, experience and personality.

On the first day of interviews for selection of ECD field team members, a very enthusiastic applicant appeared for an interview. During her interview, Amber explained that she was very keen to work in the ECD program as she felt that the only way to develop her community was by way of ensuring early childhood development for the children. Amber's positive spirit and her sense of ownership were vital factors in her selection as an ECD field team member.

Terms of Reference for ECD Field Team

After a final selection of candidates for the ECD field team has been made, TOR for the working of the field team in collaboration with the program staff should be laid down in consultation with the selected community ECD committee members. The basic principles of formation of TOR are the same as those adopted for the TOR of the committee, but with specific relation to the ECD field team members.

STEPS FOR ECD TEAM SELECTION
- *Make an announcement in the community inviting applicants*
- *List number of positions to be filled*
- *Divide number of positions into categories according to job description*
- *Assign minimum and maximum qualifications to each category*
- *Appoint people who will conduct interviews*
- *Schedule interviews*
- *Prepare evaluation criteria for interviews*
- *Conduct interviews*
- *Make final selection*

ECD Program Team Structure

There should be a clear team structure with well-defined reporting relationships. An ECD team can comprise of field and ECD Program Management Group, followed by a field coordinator with a field supervisor to assist if the program is large enough. They supervise the ECD field team and the community ECD committee. Try to have single reporting relationships within an ECD field team i.e. a member of the ECD field team reports only to one person who is supervising. Similarly, it is important for supervisors to be careful while giving tasks to members of the team they are supervising, and avoid handing out the same task to two different members of the ECD field team.

The field coordinator Maria asks two ECD field team members Zola and Abiba to visit house number 345 in Sanwal village, to inquire about the health of a child. When they reach the house they come to know that Femi was also there to ask about the health of the same child. Femi was sent by Ayesha the field supervisor.

FLOW CHART

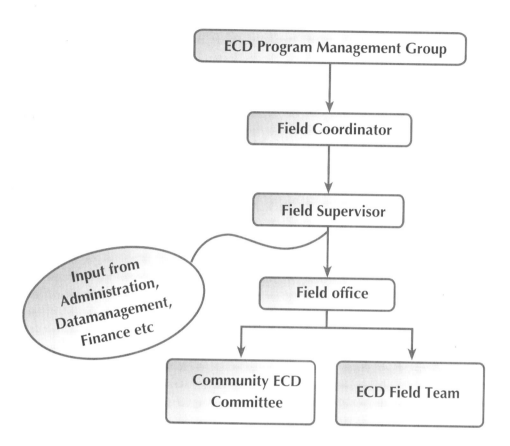

Work Plan

Maria who is the field coordinator for the ECD health education field trial had to file a report in April and only 3 days were left. She asked Shazia to give her the details regarding current activities of the team in the field, as she had to present those in the report to her supervisors. Shazia informed her that the team had completed their home visits in all areas of the community by following the program timeline and now she would be in a position to give Maria the required information in only one day. Maria was pleased with the team's work and praised the working of the team in her report.

Before starting actual field activities in an ECD field program it is vital to have a workable work plan. A work plan is used to set timelines for specific tasks related to an ECD program. Setting timelines are necessary with respect to completing different components of the program and the program as a whole on required deadlines. While setting timelines care should be taken to incorporate some room for modification. This is to accommodate an unforeseen event by which the program can get behind schedule. Therefore, a program timeline while being strict should also be flexible. There are different methods through which this is possible. "Gantt Chart" is widely used (see appendix ix).

Gantt charts can be divided into different components for ease of understanding. See appendix

I. ROWS
a. Title of the program
b. Category-wise activities list

II. COLUMNS
a. Start with serial number
b. Name of category of activity
c. Time required to complete each activity
d. Personnel responsible
e. Dates in days, weeks or months whichever is relevant to your own program

Gantt charts are planning tools that are used to plan different activities of the program according to preset timelines. Gantt charts present program planning information in a visually appealing manner by which program planning and status is visible at a glance. A Gantt chart is typically a graphic display that shows work distribution, total duration needed to complete tasks, as well as on-going status of individual tasks.

Capacity Building

The purpose of ECD capacity building is to develop personal capabilities in relation to the ECD initiative; the specific aim is that this ECD leadership will support child, family and community development in a wider social and economic development context (8).

Capacity building covers basic theoretical concepts of child development, social environment and community dynamics during training. The training also focuses on various child assessment methodologies, some of which are questionnaire-based interviews, anthropometric assessments and intellectual assessments. The training comprises classroom discussion as well as field-based exercises and activities under constant supervision and monitoring by qualified trainers. The training should be done according to a given schedule. It is important to set a total duration for the training, as well as duration of individual sessions to be conducted during the training. This enables the capacity building training given to participants to be certified. Such training enables the community ECD field team members to identify the needs and opportunities for child development applicable in the context of their own communities, and to actively pursue ECD activities in their own settings.

THEORY
It can encompass the following:
- *Child development concepts*
- *Social environment of a child*
- *Child assessment including anthropometric and intellectual assessments*
- *Observational methodology*
- *Questionnaire based interviews*
- *Communication skills*
- *Components of community based ECD programming*

PRACTICAL
Hands-on training can be provided on:
- *Assessing the level of sensory stimulation in the social environment*
- *Methods of conducting interviews*
- *Taking anthropometric measurements*
- *Collecting information on child developmental indicators*
- *Communication techniques for use in the field setting*

Baseline Assessment

Baseline community wide surveys are implemented as part of an ECD program before the application of program specific interventions (14). This is done in order to gather initial information on individual childhood, family and community developmental indicators that have been discussed in the needs assessment section in chapter 11.

> *The conventional definition of management is getting work done through people, but real management is developing people through work.*
> *-Agha Hasan Abedi*

> *Good management is the art of making problems so interesting and their solutions so constructive that everyone wants to get to work and deal with them.*
> *-Paul Hawken*

ECD field team members can collect information on child rearing practices, nutrition, health care, nurturing, and sensory stimulation available in the home environment and child growth and development indicators.

In addition, information on family and community dynamics, needs, available resources and social skills can be collected by conducting focus group discussions with caregivers, religious and community leaders, and other stakeholders.

Implementation of Community ECD Activities

Implementation of community ECD activities is possible by centre and home-based activities. Centre-based activities comprise assistance to the community ECD committee and field team members developing appropriate centre-based childcare facilities such as day care centres, educational sessions at schools or a common place of gathering, formation of self-help groups, conducting community development sessions and establishing appropriate referral systems.

In home-based activities, regular visits by the ECD field team to provide counselling and health education regarding nutrition and nurturing needs of individual children can be conducted. They can also identify growth faltering developmental delay at an early stage and can provide assistance through the referral systems set in place.

> *The environment, routines, people and activities around a child provide opportunities for spontaneous learning, which should be a feature of all early childhood learning contexts.*

HOME BASED ACTIVITIES

- *Individual information on health aspects*
- *Anthropometric assessment*
- *Monitoring of developmental indicators*
- *Door to door, provision of vaccines*
- *Reproductive health care which includes family planning advice for the parents*

CENTRE BASED ACTIVITIES

- *Day care centres*
- *Health education sessions*
- *Community meetings*
- *Education*
- *Provision of basic health care facilities*
- *Cater to referrals from the household level*
- *Special day celebrations*

> *Everyone is entitled to their own opinion, but not their own facts.*
> *-Daniel Patrick Moynihan*

Monitoring and Evaluation

Monitoring is an ongoing process of inspection and feedback on the implementation of an ECD program (9). The basic principle of monitoring is to gather information that can be used to keep a check on different components of a program; this in turn is to assess whether a program is being implemented as was planned, or not. This is important as it is concerned with the question: will the program meet its objectives?

MONITORING
Systematic process of checking and documenting ECD program performance on an ongoing basis, involving program process and outcomes

> *Thunder is good, thunder is impressive; but it is the lightning that does the work.*
> -Mark Twain

FOCUS OF MONITORING FOR ECD PROGRAMS

- Check if program resources have been mobilized
  - Maintain records (financial and other administrative records)
- Check if planned activities have been undertaken according to preset timelines
  - Maintain logbooks, arrange weekly or monthly meetings to assess progress
- Check if objectives are being met as per schedule
  - In the context of ECD this is possible by monitoring health, educational and other socio-economic indictors pertaining to ECD
- Program site visits reports
- Financial reports

Monitoring activities, with dates as to when these activities are carried out and by whom can be recorded. Documents in which monitoring information are recorded can also be mentioned. See the table below for assistance:

EVALUATION
Systematic process to assess the extent to which ECD programs meet objectives

YEAR - MONTH: MONITORING RECORD			
Date	Activity	Staff in charge	Detail

Evaluation is a systematic process to measure the effectiveness of an ECD program in achieving preset objectives (9). In the context of an ECD program evaluation, it could be seen whether the interventions implemented in the program have the desired result or not, whether those results are applicable elsewhere and if they have had an impact on child development indicators or not. Responsibilities can be designated for conducting evaluation activities. Results of an ECD program evaluation provide useful information regarding future developmental needs of the community, and the development of the next phase of the program.

Assessment of children's growth, development and learning will be part of the information needed to evaluate the program

Report Writing

A report is a document that details all the processes and activities undertaken in a program, its results, the impact the program has had on the community, and further recommendations (10). Reports are shared with all the concerned program parties, and can be used to disseminate information to a wider audience when required.

Reports are important inputs in the management and administration of a program. Reports can also be standardized to a required format suiting the needs of the program. Some components of report writing for an ECD program are:

- Background
- Historical data
- Methodology of the ECD program
- Results of the program
- Discussion

Ethical Considerations

While designing and implementing ECD community based programs, it is important to keep in mind the ethical considerations that arise. Steps should be taken to address these concerns in a just and practical manner.

There are three guiding principles under which ECD programs can be implemented in a community (11). These are:

Respect

This requires that the independence of individual members of the community be recognized. For those with diminished independence e.g. poor, pregnant women etc, it is required that they be given due protection. Respect also requires that information about community members be kept confidential.

If in one household it is observed that the developmental indicators of a child are not at par with recommended guidelines, then this information should not be shared with other households.

Beneficence

Under this principle, the ECD program team is required to "do no harm" and take necessary steps to "maximize possible benefits and minimize possible harms". When implementing an ECD program in a community, ensure that the interventions to be introduced do not have a detrimental effect on the individual and the collective social fabric of the community.

If the existing laws of the country regarding child labour are implemented in a community, it is incumbent upon the ECD program team to evaluate the effects that can result from a specific implementing action in a particular community.

Justice

All members of the community should be treated equally. The burden and benefits of an ECD program should be equally distributed within a community. Additionally an ECD program should be fair to all participating stakeholders.

Make sure that any group within the community is not marginalized due to their lack of interaction, social-economic status, caste, religion or other related factors.

The community as a whole should be taken into confidence regarding the objectives of the program. Consent from the community elders is a vital component along with individual consent from parents of children not able to give consent on their own. The parents of participating children and the community

---

Let me give you the definition of ethics: it is good to maintain life and to further life. It is bad to damage and destroy life. And this ethic, profound and universal, has the significance of a religion. It is religion.
-Albert Schweitzer

Three basic ethical principles for ECD programs
- *Respect*
- *Beneficence*
- *Justice*

Important Ethical Considerations in ECD Programs
- *Respect partial or complete refusals*
- *Disseminate information collected from the community to the stakeholders in the community*
- *Maintain confidentially*
- *Adopt system of referral for participants with malnutrition or other health disorders who are identified as persons requiring specialized care.*

> *Conventionality is not morality.*
> -Charlotte Bronte

need to be reassured that individual confidentiality will be honoured during and after the end of the program. Information collected, relating to ECD and status of the children in the community, will be disseminated to the participants and to the community as a whole.

Summary

- **ECD program management** covers overall planning and co-ordination of a program from inception to completion. Program implementation is accomplished in phases. ECD program management is a skilful job and requires coordination at different levels

- **ECD program implementation** phases begin with identification of a community, formation of a community ECD committee, selection of a field ECD team, conducting baseline surveys and implementation of home- and centre-based ECD activities in the community. A system of monitoring and evaluation should be in place for quality check and quality assurance.

- **Field Coordinator** should possess good leadership and managerial qualities that include *provision of vision, awareness of local perspectives of the community, good communication skills, ability to mobilize and encourage team members, confidence in decision-making, providing guidelines for team members' interaction with each other.*

- **Community ECD committees** should be formed by taking necessary steps to include people from different segments with relevant experience and skills to have a wider representation. For this, community mobilization can take on the shape of a community movement starting a process of communication among ECD program stakeholders and facilitating a participatory decision-making process.

- **ECD field team** should be composed of individuals who are *motivated and enthusiastic about working in the community, express genuine interest in child development, act in a positive and constructive manner, understand personal and team roles, and can maintain confidentiality.* Finally select the most appropriate person for the job, keeping in view qualifications, experience and personality.

- **Work plans,** and setting timelines for ECD programs are necessary in order to complete different components according to required deadlines. There are different methods through which this is possible. The "Gantt Chart" is widely used.

- **Capacity building** through training focuses on theoretical concepts with hands-on training. To certify capacity building training it is important that this be done according to a given schedule and structure.

- **Community ECD activities** are centre- and home-based. Examples of the former are *day care centres, educational sessions at schools or a common place of gathering and formation of self-help groups.* While the latter includes *visits by the ECD field team to provide counselling and health education regarding nutrition and nurturing needs of individual children,* such visits have the added advantage of identifying developmental weaknesses at an early stage, and can provide assistance through the referral systems set in place.

- **Essential elements of report writing** include *background, historical data, methodology and results of the program and discussion.*

- **Basic ethical principles** for ECD programs are *respect* for the individual, *beneficence* in taking necessary steps to maximize possible benefits and minimizing possible harm, and *justice* to ensure equitable access to ECD related initiatives.

The first step in the evolution of ethics is a sense of solidarity with other human beings.
-Albert Schweitzer

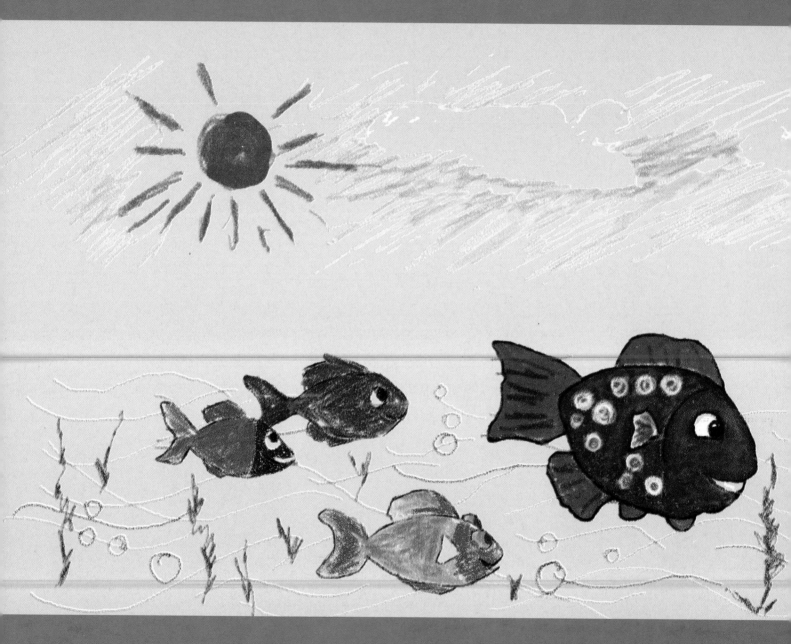

"*God gave us memory so that we might have roses in December.*
-James Matthew Barrie"

Artist:
Aliya
Age: 5 years

teaching and training

part D

teaching

And Training

Introduction

Information on child development is available from several sources such as books and journals; now even the electronic media opens unlimited opportunities to learn. It is important that such assorted knowledge should be integrated and synthesized; the internal consistency challenged, and best features put into practice. For most learners, such small pieces of knowledge remain unrelated, and they remain unable to put the complete picture together. It is important that any ECD material like this book be supplemented by teaching and training efforts.

Teaching is the usual mode for transmission of concepts into knowledge. The activity of facilitated learning of concepts can take place through lectures, seminars and other interactive sessions, and through well-written texts.

Training is the preferred mode for transmission of skills related to application of knowledge. The activity of facilitated learning of skills can take place during tutorials, workshops, and other interactive sessions, even through hands-on experience during internships.

EXPERIENTIAL LEARNING

Knowledge, skills, and abilities attained through observation, simulation, and participation that provides depth and meaning to learning by engaging the mind and body through activity, reflection, and application.
-Craig

In developing countries, most of the teaching and training for ECD discipline is conventional and instructive, the teacher being involved in one-way communication of knowledge, with the student a passive recipient of it. This unthinking learning about early child development has limited ability to relate to and extend the learning to children, caregivers and communities. Our suggestive approach for training of ECD endeavors is based on interaction between three key factors, the educator, learner, and the social environment, which provides the context. The interaction between educator and learner needs to start much by learner's communication of their needs and the educator's effort to understand the social, cultural and baseline knowledge of the learner. This will lead to mutual planning, designing and implementation of the learning process, keeping the contextual needs in perspective. In addition, this interaction process also provides experiential learning opportunity. The educator purposely exposes the learner to the practical scenarios, and provides first hand experience in the context of contemporary ECD challenges and concepts. This approach not only brings in-depth appreciation of theory but also explain the practical utility of that knowledge.

Conscious efforts need to be made by the educator and the learner to incorporate the latest learning experiences with the existing knowledge base and modification of existing knowledge base by the latest experiences. The achievement is effectively possible if theory and practice sessions innovatively integrate reflections of the learner for every ECD topic.

Rationale

Understanding of early childhood development for care and nurturance at individual level for programming and services at professional level is important to achieve success in the human development process. Especially for developing countries, ECD is relatively a new initiative, due to which there is a paucity of persons with broad-based understanding and ability to make a case for integrated care for child development. Teaching and training are one of the important ways to develop the capacity of individuals, by developing the necessary knowledge base and skills, so that each individual can play his/her role for ECD at family and community level. This demand has led us to develop this section of the book to assist caregivers to develop their knowledge and skills related to ECD.

Content

The process of providing care and supportive environment to children is learned through amalgamation of theory and practice, without creating any imbalance between them. In the previous sections, the book focused on detailed theoretical account of child development in the context of the social environment of a developing country as well as community interactions and required actions. This part of the text is primarily based on all twelve chapters, as to how each one of them can be transformed into sessions of teaching and training.

Format

Each chapter is represented first by a list of objectives for the teaching sessions; the theoretical knowledge for those objectives is discussed in detail in the specified chapter. The teaching session should be interactive and modified in accordance with the baseline knowledge level of the learner. Optimal use of audio-visual aids is recommended; in addition, special care should be given to setting and duration of settings of the session. For the training session, each chapter is followed by activities based on specified theoretical concepts to enhance experiential learning for ECD. The range of activities suggested include

- Brainstorming
- Role plays
- Group working and discussions
- Hands-on experience for child assessments
- Structured field trips for field based activities and firsthand observations.

The description of each activity includes

- **Title** of the exercise
- **Goals and objectives** to be achieved
- Suggested **Duration** of the activity
- **Trainers' preparation** for logistics and materials
- Steps of **Methodology** for the conduct of the session
- Guidelines for post activity **Discussion** session
- Possible **Variations** to conduct with changing context and learners
- Conclusion with identification of the educational **Outcome** by the learners

> *The liberally educated are those who are able to make an action out of knowledge, use knowledge to*
> - *Think*
> - *Judge*
> - *Decide*
> - *Discover*
> - *Interact, and Create*
>   *-Loacke*

Users

The knowledge and skills of Early Childhood Development are relevant and noteworthy for different groups of people such as ECD trainers, ECD services related professionals, and paraprofessionals including grassroots workers, to enable them to perform competently their professional responsibilities; other caregivers together with parents are equally relevant in order to facilitate them to play effectively their personal roles.

How to use

The concepts and activities in the book have a specific link and progression, starting from core concepts of child development, going on to child assessment and appropriate advice for growth and development, and finishing with community based initiatives to achieve holistic child development. For teaching and training purposes, the sessions should be customized by making them more culturally and linguistically appropriate.

It is important to note that it is not always necessary to use given descriptions either as a whole or in a specified sequence; contents and order may be modified according to the context and learners. In addition, ideas for teaching and training are evocative, not exhaustive. Other material sources can be searched for and incorporated, in order to customize session according to the learner's need.

Teaching and training sessions should follow the actively participatory and experiential learning approach. The contents are organized to conduct group sessions, but at individual level, it can still be a valid educational tool. In that case, the individual should personally monitor and appreciate the achievement of learning outcomes.

Conclusion

The purpose is not to provide specific prescriptions of tailor-made steps for ECD caregivers and service providers for direct application at family and community levels. The intention is to enhance knowledge, skills and perceptions; and motivate integrated and joint actions by all those who do care for children.

The overall objectives of this part of the book can be summarized as:
- Awareness of age appropriate growth and development of children
- Understanding of physical, social and emotional requirements during early childhood
- Identification of local socio-cultural perceptions and practices which affect child development
- Development of skills for scientific assessment of child's growth and development
- Ability of scientific advice given to caregivers to prevent the child's growth from faltering and developmental delay
- Orientation of child development challenges at community level
- Capacity to develop community based initiatives, for creating conducive opportunities for holistic child development by involving all caregivers including service providers.

chapter one

FUNDAMENTALS OF CHILD DEVELOPMENT

Learning Objectives

By the end of the session, participants would be able to:

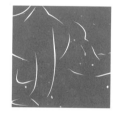

- Define human development

- List various phases of human development

- Enumerate and describe various domains of early childhood development

- Identify and understand various critical factors for child development

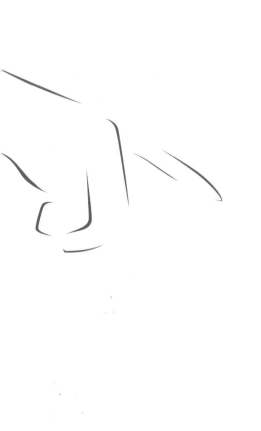

Activity 1: *Brainstorming*

Title: Issues and challenges of early childhood development

Goal: To develop understanding of important categories of factors effecting child development, and the ability to address them within their local context.

Objectives:
To identify and discuss problems and solutions, at least for the following factors for their respective community.
● Health and nutrition
● Caregiver's attitude
● Physical and social environment

Duration: 2 hours

Trainer Preparation:
● Flipcharts and markers.
● Enough space for seating small groups, so that the working group remains uninterrupted by adjacent groups' discussions.

Method:
● Divide the participants into small groups of five members each.
● Distribute markers & flip charts to each group.
● Provide them with an earlier briefing, so that they come prepared with thoughts and comments regarding major problems and issues affecting child development of this under 6 years age group. This task should be completed through group discussion, in a given time of 45 minutes.
● Guide them to draw a sketch of a child in the middle of the chart; close to this picture, they should draw a balloon in which they should note down one major problem, affecting children of this age group.
● They should then reflect on the consequences of this problem.
● They should draw a new balloon, enter in it another problem and link it to the first problem. They should continue drawing and linking other balloons representing the consequences of those problems.
● When a whole chain of balloons has been created in this way they should reflect on how and where the chain of negative consequences can be broken.
● In the end, the small groups should sum up their discussion and share it with the other groups and facilitators.

Questions for discussion:
● The facilitator can ask about the range of the caregivers involved during child development and how each of them can contribute to address these issues and challenges.

Learning outcome:
● This activity will help participants discuss and share their views regarding child development and to realize that others share the same concerns. This interaction will enhance their ability to carry out situation analysis and identification of solutions to challenges regarding child development within their own context.

VARIATIONS:
● *Individuals can be asked to identify the problems faced by children in their respective homes, they can then combine these factors at group level.*
● *Each group can be assigned any one year of early childhood, from birth to 6 years. This will help to discuss the specific problems and challenges of each year during the early childhood phase.*

Activity 2: *Role Play*

Title: Child development milestones

Goal: To develop the ability to understand that child development has various domains.

Objectives:
To identify age-appropriate child growth and developmental milestones:
- Physical growth
- Mental development
- Emotional development
- Social development

Duration: 2 hours

Trainer Preparation:
- Copies of growth and developmental milestone chart. (see appendix).
- Preferably in a closed space, as some of participants may not feel comfortable performing their roles in an open space.

Method:
- The participants may be divided into small groups.
- Growth and developmental milestone charts can be distributed to each participant.
- Brief participants to nominate two members from each group by consensus decision; these representatives can play the role of primary caregivers. Each group should be given 15 minutes, and they will have to perform their roles in front of all the participants.
- During the act, players will discuss their children's milestones and related joys and apprehensions, the remaining participants observe the content of verbal as well as non-verbal communication of the players. Any observation or comments regarding the personality of the players should be discouraged.

Questions for discussion:
After every role-play, the facilitator should generate discussion on the milestones considered in the role-play.
- Ask the participant if the players have correctly mentioned age-appropriate milestones, and ask what else can be added to get a comprehensive view of the child's developmental status.
- In addition, discuss whether the reasons for joy or apprehension were appropriate or not.
- What could be the possible solution in response to the apprehensions of the caregivers?
- The session should be summarised by asking the participants to comments on the salient features they have understood regarding the various domains of child development.

Learning outcome:
- This activity will provide the opportunity for trainers to understand and experience the conventional roles, responsibilities and expectations of different types of caregivers. In addition, such an activity helps identify age-appropriate milestones for growth and development of the child.

> **VARIATION**
> *Individuals in a group can be asked to play the role of different type of caregivers, such as mother, father, sibling, relatives and childcare service providers e.g. health, education etc.*

Supportive considerations

- During early childhood, the brain gains weight, partly due to an increase in the number of brain cells, and partly due to the growth of "connections" between cells and different parts of the brain. Without these connections we cannot think, and it is through these connections that learning begins. The connections in a newborn child start to form a network: when the child becomes interested in something it makes a mental effort and some of his / her senses are stimulated. So from the moment of birth, the brain is continuously conditioned by the sensory experiences of sounds, sights, touches, smells and tastes to make more connections. It is important that sight, sound, memory and motor skills move forward together, for mental growth to proceed. The intellect is dependent on the senses and body movement for the baby to understand what is going on around him / her.

- This concept needs emphasis, to stress that child development occurs in holistic fashion and not in isolation.

- It is important to relate the concept and domains of child development with every module throughout ECD training.

- Continuous reinforcements of concepts of child development will be needed, and would be an important aid to learning charts of milestones of children from age 1 month to 72 months.

- Generate discussion about the given scenario. In order to bring participants to the topic of Child Development with a focus on Early Child Development and its milestones, throw a significant question to the participants, such as:
  - *What do you think mothers usually discuss among themselves regarding their children?*

- After seeking their attention through discussion, explain to them the topic of Child Development.

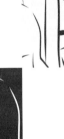

chapter two

SOCIAL ENVIRONMENT

Learning Objectives

By the end of the session, participants would be able to:

- Define the social environment that affects growth and development during early childhood.

- List the various senses, which receive stimulation from the environment.

- Identify some of the critical elements of the social environment.

- Understand the significance of the social environment in relation to early childhood development.

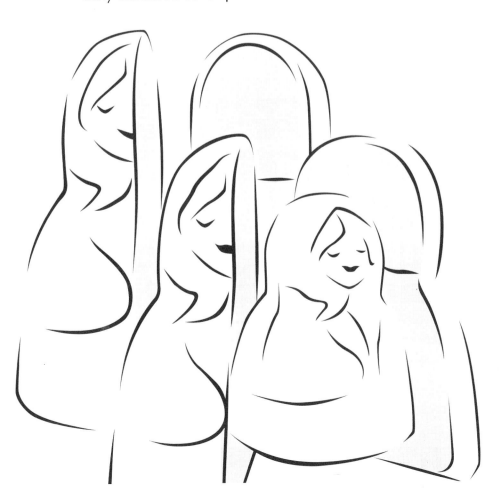

Activity 1: *Group Activity*

Title: Sensory stimulation to the child

Goal: To develop the significance of sensory stimulation to the child

Objective:
- To identify possible stimulation mechanisms related to the five senses (hearing, touch, smell, taste and sight).

Duration: 2 hours

Trainer Preparation:
- Note pad, pencil and eraser.
- Different items to be used for sensory stimulation (fruits, toys, and other daily use items).

Method:
- Divide participants into five groups.
- Distribute five items to each group.
- Brief participants on observation of different items and recording the senses that can be evoked by each item.
- Give participants 30 minutes to complete and record their observations.
- Ask each group to summarize the information compiled and make its own presentation.

Questions for discussion:
- By discussing the concept of sensory stimulation and the mechanisms involved, the facilitator can demonstrate how one object can evoke multiple senses. Ask the participants if they consider it necessary to stimulate children. Ask the participants about the items they would use to stimulate children, in order to elicit specific senses.

Learning outcome:
- Participants will learn that sensory stimulation is an ongoing process, and is achievable irrespective of socio-economic status without difficulty. They will also appreciate that a single object can stimulate multiple senses simultaneously.

Activity 2: *Role Playing*

Title: Social environment during ECD

Goal: To develop an understanding of the significance and interaction of critical elements of social environment in ECD.

Objectives:
To identify critical elements relating to child environment such as:
- Internal relationships
- External relationships
- External services

> **VARIATION**
> *Ask the groups of participants to observe the surrounding environment of the room and look for items that can elicit a particular sense. Each group can be asked to make observations for one stimulatory sense.*

- Socio-cultural and Political context
- Significant life events

Duration: 2 hours

Trainer Preparation (Materials):
- Note pad, pencil and eraser.

Method:
- Begin by dividing participants into five groups.
- Brief them on how to nominate two members from their particular group who will play the assigned role.
- Role-playing should be after consensus has been reached by the group participants; observations about personalities of the players should be discouraged.
- Assign one domain of social environment to each of the following groups:
  - Group one – Internal relationships (e.g. Father returns home in the evening and interacts with his child).
  - Group two – External relationships (e.g. Teacher is talking to children in the classroom about always telling the truth).
  - Group three – External services (e.g. Child is brought to the clinic of a doctor to be vaccinated and is resisting).
  - Group four – Socio-cultural & Political context (e.g. Community meeting to discuss opening of a new school for girls in the community).
  - Group five – Significant life events (e.g. Expressions of a four-year-old child on the birth of his/her sibling).
- The remaining participants will be required to make observations on the role-plays.
- Ask each group to summarize their observations and make separate presentations after each respective role-play.

Questions for discussion:
- The facilitator can ask participants about the concept of a social environment and its critical elements. A discussion on how these critical elements influence a child development can also be generated. Participants can also be asked about how primary care givers would function in different critical elements of a given social environment.

Learning outcome:
- Participants will develop understanding about the fact that critical elements of the social environment are also relevant to their environment. They will develop the skill to relate critical elements and influences to each other.

Activity 3: *Field Visit*

Title: Environment appraisal in the context of ECD

Goal: To develop appraisal skills for the child related environment

Objectives:
To appreciate the differences in child related environment with respect to:

- Caregiver involvement
- Age appropriate expectations of child development and behaviour status
- Order and organization
- Assortment of interactions
- Learning opportunities

Duration: 4 hours

Trainer Preparation:
- Note pad, pencil and eraser.
- Arrangement of logistics before time for instance, venue (school, household), transport, advance information to the concerned people.

VARIATION
Similar visits can be arranged to a play area and a clinic for appraisal of the relevant of child-related environment.

Method:
- Divide participants into two groups.
- Assign specific tasks to groups as under:
  - ☐ Group one – Observe a living room setting in a household.
  - ☐ Group two – Observe a classroom setting in a school.
- Ask participants to write down their observations in relation to the particular social environment in each field setting.
- Participants can make presentations after they have returned and summarized their observations.
- Differences in child related environment domains in the two settings should be discussed.

Questions for discussion:
- The facilitator will ask the participants as to which environment is more conducive for child development, especially for learning. The facilitator will also ask the participants to reflect upon the possible causes for differences.

Learning outcome:
- Participants will develop necessary appraisal skills for assessment of child related environments.
- Participants will also learn to appreciate that each environmental domain has its particular strengths and weaknesses with respect to influencing the child.
- Importance of providing a variety of environments related to caregiver involvement, age appropriate expectations of child development and behaviour status, order and organization, assortment of interactions, and learning opportunities for children will also be understood.

Supportive considerations
- Social environment provides the opportunities to use the senses, and the child learns from the environment by using all his senses; therefore, participants should know about all the senses and how they work together.

- Learners should have some basic knowledge about physical, mental, social and emotional development, so they can understand the importance of the social environment in the child's holistic development.

- It is important for the trainer to define the environmental context of child development with common examples of participant communities; the use of charts or diagrams would be helpful.

- The facilitator can give an assignment to the learner to carefully note children's social environment and then narrate their observations.

Supportive considerations

Ecological System

In literature, the concept of a social environment which influences child development is referred to as "The Ecology of Human Development." In this text, the concept and terminologies have been adapted to address the needs of a wider audience. However, a brief overview of the original concept is given below for reference purposes.

A. The Micro System (Internal Relationships)

The innermost level of the ecological system is the micro system, which refers to the activities and interaction patterns in a child's immediate surroundings. It is important to note that at this level, all relationships are bi-directional, i.e. the adults affect the child's behavior, personality and skills, which in turn affects adult behavior.

B. The Meso System (External Relationships)

The meso system deals with the interconnection between the child's immediate settings such as home, school, daycare center and play area that foster child development. A child's progress at a daycare center or in school does not just depend on the activities that take place in class, but also on the parent's involvement in his/her school life. Similarly, parent-child and caregiver-child relationships are likely to support development when there are links in the form of visits and exchange of information between home and child-care setting.

C. The Exo System (External Services)

This refers to the setting that does not contain children, but affects their experiences in immediate settings. These may be formal organizations such as parents' work place or health and welfare services in the community, and informal parents' social networks as well.

D. The Macro System (Socio-Cultural and Political Context)

The macro system consists of cultural values, laws and customs. The priority that the macro system gives to a child's need affects the support they receive at the inner level of the environment.

E. The Chrono System (Significant Life Events)

This system deals with the concept that the environment is not a static force which affects people in a uniform way, it is, on the other hand, ever changing. Important life events, such as the birth of a sibling, entering school, moving to a new neighbourhood or family conflict etc. modify the relationship between children and their environment, producing new conditions that affect development. In addition, the timing of environmental change also affects its impact.

chapter three

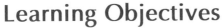

GENERAL GUIDELINES FOR CHILD ASSESSMENT

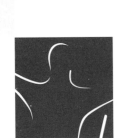

Learning Objectives

By the end of the session, participants would be able to:

- Define child assessment.

- Identify need for child assessment.

- Enlist various precautions for child assessment.

- Describe strategies for rapport building with caregiver and young child.

- Define child's temperament.

- Enlist salient characteristics of temperament.

- Describe steps of child's assessment.

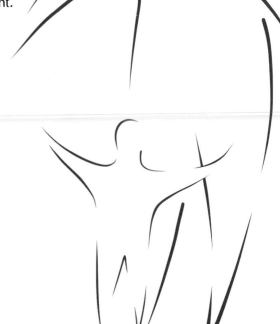

Activity 1: *Brainstorming*

Title: Rapport Building

Goal: To develop an understanding of the changing needs of assessment, with respect to a child's age.

Objectives:
To identify various ways of rapport building with children of different ages in a similar setting.
- A 2-year-old child
- A 6-year-old child

Duration: 2 hours

Trainer Preparation:
- Note pad, pencil and eraser.
- Flipchart and marker.
- Sufficient seating space for small groups, so that any one group's working remains undisturbed by adjacent groups' discussions.

Method:
- Divide the participants into two groups.
- Explain to group one a scenario of a 2-year-old child playing with toys in his home; explain the same scenario to group two with a 6-year-old child.
- Give a flipchart to each group, and ask them to write down the ways they think could be used for rapport building with children of that age group.
- Give them 30 minutes to complete this group activity.
- Ask them to share those brainstormed ideas with the rest of the participants in the large group.

Questions for discussion:
- Facilitator could ask about the differences in rapport building with children of different ages.
- He/she can ask about perceived hindrances with respect to establishing the rapport that participants feel.
- He or she can ask about the process and consideration for rapport building with children.

Learning outcome:
This activity will help the participants to come up with possible ways of rapport building among children of various ages.

VARIATIONS
- *Groups can be given different scenarios such as playground, school or day care center.*
- *Rapport building can be focused on children of various ages, sex, and socio-economic status.*
- *Brainstorming could be done on the rapport building with the caregivers, like father, mother, and grandmothers etc.*

Activity 2: *Brainstorming*

Title: Child Assessment

Goal: To provide an opportunity to understand child assessment

Objectives:
To identify and discuss the precautions for child assessment at least on the following topics:
- Test materials.

- Testing conditions.
- Physical health of the child.

Duration: 2 hours

Trainer Preparation:
- Note pad, pencil and eraser.
- Flipchart and marker.
- Sufficient seating space for small groups, so that the group which is working remains undisturbed by adjacent groups' discussions.

Method:
- Divide participants into three groups.
- Assign the following topics to each group:
    - Test materials
    - Testing conditions
    - Physical health of the child
- Ask the group to brainstorm and come up with the precautions for child assessment related to the respective topic.
- In the end, ask each group to summarize their discussion and make a presentation.

Questions for discussion:
- At the end of each group presentation the facilitator could ask questions about the importance of observing precautions during assessment with respect to the topic of discussion.
- He or she can encourage them to share their views on the effect of not taking precautionary measures during child's assessment.

Learning outcome:
- This activity will enable the participant to have a clear understanding of the need of preparations prior to a child's assessment.
- It will help them to learn about the concept of standardization for child assessment.

VARIATION
This activity can be performed to understand specific assessment requirements, needs of intellectual and emotional assessment, and psychomotor development status.

Activity 3: *Group Activity*

Title: Child's Temperament

Goal: To develop an understanding of the child's temperament and its effect on rapport building.

Objectives:
To identify various ways of rapport building with respect to temperament of:
- Easy children
- Slow to warm up children
- Difficult children

Duration: 2 hours

Trainer's Preparation:

- Small pieces of card.
- Flipchart and markers.
- Sufficient seating space for small groups, so that the group working remains undisturbed by adjacent groups' discussions.

Method:
- Divide participants into three groups with respect to child's temperament; for instance, group one will focus on easy children, group two on slow to warm up children, and group three on children with difficult temperament.
- Give small cards to each member of each group to write whatever ways he or she thinks for rapport building can be established according to specific characteristics of temperament.
- Then ask each participant to share his/her thoughts with the rest of the participants in their respective groups and write them on a flip chart.
- After this, ask each group to share their ideas with the participants of the remaining groups.

Questions for Discussion:
- The facilitator can generate discussion on the group reflections, and can relate it with the various concepts of child temperament associated with activity level, approach, task persistence etc.
- He or she can encourage participants to think about whether any importance had been given to the child's temperament, while assessing the child; and to think about how rapport was built in children of differing temperament.
- The facilitator asks the group to reflect on awareness of child's temperament for better child-caregiver relationship.

Learning outcomes:
- This activity will highlight the importance and understanding of the child's temperament.
- It will give them the ability to learn various ways of rapport building according to the temperament of the child.

VARIATION
Each group can be asked to share their views on rapport building with children of specific temperament type, of differing gender and ages.

Supportive considerations
General points to maintain the rapport with younger children

- It is necessary to be careful that instructions for the assessment are the same for all the children being assessed, because inconsistency in instructions could lead to erroneous results.

- It is essential for an assessor to keep verbal direction short, simple and clear; so that the child easily understands what the trainee wants him/ her to do.

- First give the instruction, demonstrate if appropriate, and then present material to the child so that he/ she is able to pay attention when given directions, and also during demonstration.

- Use a game format for instance, "your turn" / "my turn" to maintain the relationship during assessment.

- Sometimes it is better to allow the child to take the lead and play with the materials in a non-directional way. When the child is attentive, the assessor can structure the activity to get the required information.

- The assessor can use attention-getting phrases like "watch me" and "are you ready" etc. before the child begins the tasks.

- If an assessor feels that he/she will have to come again to assess the child, then on departing, he/she can tell the child that "I will see you soon and we will play again." so that the reappearance of the assessor does not make the child uneasy.

- Above all, a child of any age should perceive the assessment as a positive experience. A relaxed and playful approach to the child conveys to him/ her that evaluation will be an enjoyable experience.

Supportive considerations

Assessor's Characteristics

It is generally observed that assessment results also vary according to the assessor's characteristics. Personality characteristics can be depicted in terms of:

- **Communication skills**
  Ability to initiate communication with children is vital; otherwise, this may lead to a **communication gap between the assessor and the child being assessed.**

- **Tolerance and Affection**
  Ability to tolerate the child's negative behaviour towards the assessment, and gradually gaining the child's confidence.

- **Experience**
  It also makes things easier for the assessor if he/ she knows the ways to handle situations tactfully for a smoother assessment process and good results.

chapter four

NUTRTITION, GROWTH AND ANTHROPOMETRY

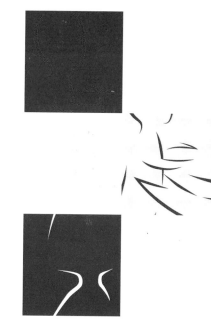

Learning Objectives

By the end of the session, participants would be able to:

- Define the term nutrition.

- Describe the concept of a healthy diet.

- Describe nutritional needs during pregnancy and lactation.

- Describe nutritional needs during childhood.

- Discuss various factors affecting nutrition.

- Define the concept of anthropometry.

- List steps of anthropometric measurements of a child.

- Explain the plotting and interpretation of anthropometric measurements on growth charts.

- Describe significance of nutritional counselling to a mother regarding her own diet and that of her child.

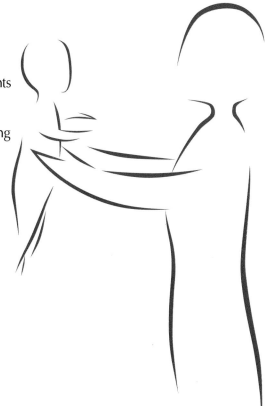

Activity 1: *Brain storming*

Title: Nutritional needs during pregnancy and early childhood

Goal: To develop the understanding of importance of nutrition with reference to particular phases of life.

Objective:
To identify and discuss problems and solution, regarding the nutritional requirements of 0-6 years old children and pregnant women in their respective communities.

Duration: 2 hours

VARIATION
Individuals can be asked to find out the nutritional needs of each year of life until 6 years of age i.e. age appropriate balanced diet.

Trainer Preparation:
- Flipcharts and markers.
- Enough space for seating small groups, so that any one group's working remains undisturbed by adjacent groups' discussions.

Method:
- Divide the participants into small groups of five members each.
- Distribute markers & flipcharts to each group.
- Brief them so that each group of participant takes one food group and lists the sources of that particular food group available in their area.
- Ask them to describe the changing requirements of their respective food group with respect to pregnancy and childhood.
- They should then reflect on the consequences of malnutrition during pregnancy and childhood.
- This task should be achieved through group discussion in a given time of 45 minutes.
- In the end small groups should sum up their discussion and share it with other groups and facilitators.

Questions for discussion:
- The facilitator can ask the participants about challenges faced in the community for the availability of food for the expectant mothers and children.

Learning outcome:
- It is important for participants to realise the nutritive value of locally available food; they should come up with the best possible ways to meet the nutritional needs of the vulnerable population groups within available resources.

Activity 2: *Role play*

Title: Malnutrition in the context of pregnancy and early childhood

Goal: To make the participants understand the effects and consequences of malnutrition during critical periods of life.

Objectives:
To identify and discuss the problem of malnutrition and its solution, at least for the following groups of population for their respective community:

- Pregnant women
- Children (0-6 years of age)

Duration: 2 hours

Trainer Preparation:
- Flipcharts and markers.
- Preferably in a closed space, as some of participants may not feel comfortable performing their roles in an open space.

Method:
- Begin by dividing participants into two groups.
- Distribute flipcharts and markers to each group.
- Brief them on how to nominate two members from their particular group who will play the assigned role.
- Select the nominated participants from group one to play the role of a pregnant woman and a worker from social services. From group two, also select the nominated participants who will assume the role of a caregiver and a worker from social services.
- Give them two different scenarios related to maternal malnutrition and child malnutrition:
  (i)   A pregnant woman is very weak and is not gaining weight. Upon discussion with the worker from social services, it becomes evident that she has restricted her diet by considering certain foods 'hot' in their intrinsic quality and therefore harmful.
  (ii) Caregiver of an 18 months old child, who is not given any food except breast milk, is very much concerned about repeated sickness and poor growth of the child; she/he discusses this problem with the worker from social services.
- Give each group a role-play time of 30 minutes.
- The remaining participants will be required to make observations on the role-play.
- Ask participant to summarize their observations regarding both the role-plays.

Questions for discussion:
- At the end of the role-play obtain feedback from the rest of the participants. Also discuss what are the reasons, solutions and challenges for malnutrition among pregnant women and children (0-6 years) at the level of:
  □   Internal relationships (how families can contribute in the proper nutrition of pregnant women, and children 0-6 years of age).
  □   External relationships (how neighbourhood, childcare centres, and schools can contribute to the proper nutrition of pregnant women, and children 0-6 years of age).
  □   External services (how community health services, social welfare services, can contribute to the proper nutrition of pregnant women, and children 0-6 years of age).
  □   Socio-cultural and political context (how the government can give strong political support to mother and child nutritional policies).
- The session should be summarised by asking the participants to comment on salient features they have learnt about various reasons and solutions for the problem of malnutrition in pregnant women and children.

Learning Outcome:
- The participants will learn the causes of malnutrition in the context of pregnancy and childhood.
- They will be able to identify malnutrition related challenges, and will find the solutions, keeping their own resources in mind.

Activity 3: *Group working and discussions*

Title: Making a local-events calendar

Goal: To determine the age of the children by relating it to some specific events occurring during their time of birth.

Objective:

To develop the skills for determination of a child's age, whose date of birth is not known as happens in developing countries where home deliveries take place and birth records are not maintained.

Duration: 2 hours

Trainer Preparation (Materials):

- Gregorian calendars of the current year and the last 6 years at least.
- Local calendar such as Hijri/Vikrami (Hindi) etc. of the current year and the last three years.
- Flipcharts and markers.
- Enough space for seating of small groups, so that the group working remains uninterrupted by adjacent groups' discussions.

Method:

- Divide the participants into small groups of five members each.
- Distribute Markers, Flipcharts, Gregorian and local calendar e.g. Hijri/Vikrami (as appropriate to that community) to each group.
- Explain to participants that a local events calendar shows all the dates on which important events took place during the past 3-5 year period. It may show different seasons, months, and phases of moon, local festivals and events in the agricultural cycle. These types of events remain in the memory of local people who otherwise are not literate, and may not be able to tell the exact dates of birth of their children. The following example could be helpful in understanding the concept:
- For example, on April 12, 2007, the participants happen to meet a caregiver who does not know the age of his/her child. Nor is there any documentary proof (e.g. birth certificate, vaccination card) that could help in assessing the child's age. The caregiver says that since the child was born at home, no birth certificate exists, the vaccination card is also lost. In that case, the participant can ask the caregiver to remember any particular event pertinent to their setting, close to which the child was born. If the caregiver says that the child was born two days after the annual religious festival of last year, then looking at the local events calendar one can figure out the exact age of a child.
- Brief the participants to come up with important events that happened in their community during the last one year by making a local events calendar.
- This task should be achieved through group discussion in a given time of 45 minutes.
- When all groups have completed the activity ask them to share their work with all training participants in plenary.

Questions for discussion:

- The facilitator can ask about different occasions/events that might have been missed by the participants.
- Discuss the individual problems faced by the participants preparing a local events calendar.

VARIATION

Individuals can be asked to find a child in their home or neighbourhood who has a birth record of the content of they are ignorant. They should try to find out the age of the child with the help of a local events calendar first, and then, they should compare that with the child's actual date of birth as given in the birth record. In this way, they can assess how close they are to estimating the correct age with the help of a local events calendar.

Various Events in a year
Religious festival for Muslims (Eid-uz-Zoha)
Important religious day (Ashura)
New Year festival for Persians and Parsis (Navroze)
End of harvest (Holi)
Horse and cattle show
Religious festival for Christians (Easter)
Prophet Muhammad's (PBUH) birthday
Religious festival for Hindus (Devali)
Religious festival for Muslims (Eid-ul-fitr)
Religious festival for Christians (Christmas)

Learning outcome:

- Use of local-events calendar is a simple and non-expensive way of calculating the approximate age of the child. However, it is of low reliability. This exercise will help the participants to include the children for growth assessment, who otherwise cannot be provided meaningful measurements because of inability to compare with age- specific standards.

Activity 4: *Group working*

Title: Performing anthropometry

Goal: To develop the skills for performing anthropometric measurements to assess the growth and health of children.

Objectives:

To help participants to take correctly anthropometric measurements of:

- Height
- Weight
- Head circumference

Duration: 2 hours

Trainer Preparation:

- Infant weighing scale.
- Bath room scale.
- Stadiometer (length/height measuring board).
- Measuring tape.
- Rulers.
- Note pads, pencils and erasers.
- Enough space for keeping the scales and for performing anthropometry.
- Permission in advance from the school to be visited, and for arrangement of transport.

Method:

- This activity has two steps; the first step should be conducted in the training room and the second step in a nearby school.

VARIATION

The participants can perform the same activity for infants and small children in their neighbourhood after obtaining informed consent of the parents.

- Divide the participants into groups of 2 members each.
- Distribute pencils, erasers, rulers and note pads to the participants.
- Ask the participants to take anthropometric measurements of each other.
- The participants should be taken to the nearby school.
- Arrange the height and weight measurement scales at an appropriate place in the school with the guidance of school administration staff.
- The participants should again be divided into groups of two members each, and should perform anthropometric measurements on each other of height, weight and head circumference by standard techniques and should record these on note pads.

Questions for discussion:
- The facilitator can ask about the experience of the whole activity including the process, and problems etc. Summarize the session by debriefing important steps for anthropometric assessments.

Learning outcome:
- The hands-on experience of taking anthropometric measurements would enhance the understanding of challenges of anthropometric assessment at community level.
- The participants will get an understanding of the measurement scales, and will learn the skills of accurately performing anthropometric assessment.

Activity 5: *Group working*

Title: Filling and interpretation of Growth Chart

Goal: Making the participants evaluate the age-appropriate growth of a child

Objectives:
To help the participants so that after completing anthropometric assessments they should be able to:
- Plot the growth parameters on the growth chart
- Interpret the plotting on the growth chart

Duration: 2 hours

Trainer Preparation:
- Blank growth charts.
- Note pad, pencils and erasers.
- Rulers.
- Anthropometric data (photocopies).

Method:
- Divide the participants in groups of two members each.
- Provide a blank growth chart (weight-for-age type) to each group and give them the information mentioned below to plot the weight measurements on the growth chart and interpret it as well:

A boy named Adam was born in June, 2004. He was weighed at different months following his birth. His weight and month of weighing is given below:

Year	Month	Weight	Additional Information
2005	June	3.0 Kg	
	July	4.0 Kg	
	Aug	4.5 Kg	
	Sep	5.5 Kg	
	Oct	6.0 Kg	
	Nov	-	Weight was not taken as the child went to aunt's village
	Dec	-	
2006	Jan	7.0 Kg	
	Feb	-	Had measles
	March	6.5 Kg	Had diarrhoea
	Apr	6.0 Kg	Advised special nutrition care
	May	6.5 Kg	
	June	7.5 Kg	
	Sep	9.0 Kg	
	Oct	10.5 Kg	
	Dec	11.5 Kg	
2007	Jan	11.5 Kg	Stopped breast feeding
	Feb	11.5 Kg	
	Apr	10.5 Kg	
	June	12.0 Kg	

Dates used are examples

- Ask the participants to put dots in the appropriate columns for the weights given above and join these dots by a line.
- This task should be achieved through group discussion in a given time of 30 minutes.

Questions for discussions:
- The facilitator can ask the participants to keep in mind the additional information given in the table and to answer the following questions: (examples are given below):

a) How old was Adam in January 2005 and July 2006?
(Answer: 7 months old, and 2 years and 1 month in 2006).

b) What does the growth line show between June to December 2004?
(Answer: Normal growth).

c) What does the growth line show between March to June 2005?
(Answer: as the direction of the line is downwards, it indicates that the child is losing weight and is malnourished).

d) What advice should have been given to Adam's mother in March 2005?
(Answer: as the growth line is going downwards, the caregiver should have been asked to pay special attention to his diet).

e) What does the growth line show between September to December 2005?
(Answer: accelerated growth as the direction of the line is upward; means that the child is gaining weight).

VARIATION
The participants can perform the same activity for length for age, height for age, and head circumference for age.

- After 45 minutes, ask each group to share their answers.
- Make corrections if a group has not written the answers correctly, and discuss the concepts again.

Learning outcome:
- By plotting the different weights of the child, the participants will be able to find out fluctuating patterns of growth and will be more confident in doing the nutritional counselling and identification of children in need of referral.

Supportive Considerations

Field Training

The participants should be taken to a community, which resembles the community in which actual anthropometric measurements would be conducted. This will help trainees to realize the problems they could encounter in the actual field, and would help them to understand local norms and culture.

chapter five

INTELLECTUAL ASSESSMENT

Learning Objectives

By the end of the session, participants would be able to:

- Define intelligence and the domains of intelligence.

- List the factors which enhance intelligence.

- List the importance of being intelligent.

- List different intelligence measures.

- Highlight the significance of intellectual assessment in relation to ECD.

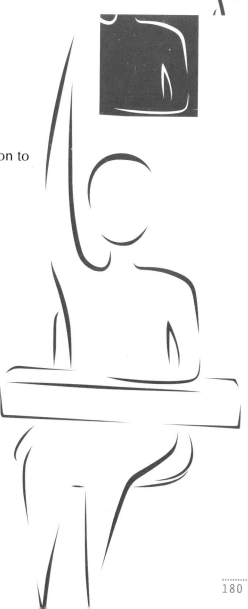

Activity 1: *Field Visit*

Title: Intellectual assessment of the child

Goal: To develop the understanding and ability to perform a child's intellectual assessment.

Objectives:
To administer the tool of intellectual assessment at least for the following domains:
- Curiosity
- Psychomotor development
- Emotional intelligence

Duration: 4 hours

Trainer Preparation (Materials):
- AKU tool for intellectual assessment (see appendix).
- Note pad, pencil and eraser.
- Arrangement of logistics before time, for instance, venue (day care centre), visit timing, transport, advance information to the administration of the day care centre.

Method:
- Visit a day care centre where children of specific age groups are available.
- Ask the participant to start the assessment by keeping all ways of rapport building in mind.
- Ask them to note down all the assessment results and observations while conducting the assessment session.
- Make sure that instructions for the assessment are the same for all children.

Questions for discussion:
- The facilitator could generate a discussion about the precautions and assessment procedure they carried out, and can encourage participants to express the problems they had during the session with respect to child assessment.
- The facilitator can express the practical experience of a child's intellectual assessment with the various domains of intelligence.
- At the end of the discussion, the facilitator can even ask them to come up with various solutions to handle the problems they might have during the child assessment.

Learning outcome:
- This activity will enable them to have a hands-on experience related to the child's intellectual assessment.
- It will give them experience in handling challenges faced due to individual variations in the temperament of children during intellectual assessment.

Activity 2: *Role-play*

Title: Understanding of Learning Styles

Goal: To develop the ability to understand and appreciate various learning styles of children.

Objectives:
To identify and describe the following learning styles of children:
- Auditory learning style
- Visual learning style
- Kinaesthetic learning style

Duration: 2 hours

Trainer Preparation:
- Note pad, pencil and eraser.
- Low cost-no cost materials like old news papers, sticks etc. that can be used as props.
- Conduct roleplay preferably in a closed space, as some of participants may not feel comfortable performing their roles in an open space.

Method:
- Divide the participants into three groups for role-play, one group for auditory learning, the second for the visual and third for the kinaesthetic learning style.
- Provide them a scenario to act on. For auditory learning group, a classroom situation can be explained where the teacher is taking a class, and some children are listening to her with great interest while others are writing, talking or even sleeping. Similarly, for the visual group in a class where the teacher is explaining a life cycle process, some children are drawing and writing about the life cycle, while others are listening or talking. In the same way for kinaesthetic learning a situation can be depicted where the teacher has taken the children out to the garden to explain to them the process of growth of plants, and some children are moving about and exploring the plants while others are listening.
- Give them 15 minutes to plan and design their roles and props for the play.
- Ask them to role-play in front of the remaining participants for 5 minutes for each play.

Questions for discussion:
- The facilitator can generate discussion at the end of each role-play session, and can ask for the participants' feedback.
- Generate discussion on the conceptual understanding of the various learning styles and the role of a conducive environment in the enhanced intellectual status of children.
- Participants could be encouraged to reflect on their feelings about the role they played, and share their views with other participants.

Learning outcome:
- This activity will help participants to have a clear understanding of different learning styles.
- It will enable them to understand the needs of children with a specific predominant learning style.
- It will let them come up with thoughts on providing a facilitating environment that will enhance children's learning.

Supportive Considerations
- During training it is important to explore the understanding of learners about the concept of intelligence; it is a prerequisite for the tool's usage to focus on the aspects related to rapport building and precautions for assessment; for this intensive training is required.

- Before initiating activities, it is prerequisite for the learners to refer to the sections on Observational Methodology and Child Assessment.

VARIATION
This activity could be used as the role-play with different caregivers in terms of their perception and understanding of various learning styles of children.

chapter six

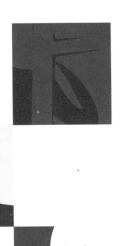

OBSERVATIONAL METHODOLOGY

Learning Objectives

By the end of the session, participants would be able to:

- Define observation of a child.

- Define the process of observation.

- List various factors involved in standardization of observation.

- List some child development related aspects that are worth observing.

- Define parenting.

- Describe conceptual domains of parenting.

- Identify parental styles in the context of conceptual domains.

- Define mechanisms to discipline a child for desirable behaviour: reinforcement and punishment.

- Describe significance of play during ECD.

- List age appropriate range of play types during early childhood.

- Understand the significance of observational methodology in relation to ECD.

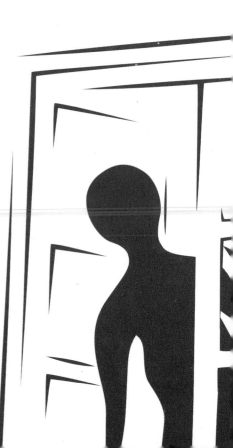

Activity 1: Field Visit

Title: Observation of children's behaviour in a real setting

Goal: To develop the skill of observing children.

Objectives:
To observe the level of physical activity of children in different settings, e.g.:
- Classroom.
- Playground.

Duration: 4 hours

Trainer Preparation:
- Note pad, pencil and eraser.
- Arrangement of logistics before time, for instance, venue, transport, advance information to the school administration.

Method:
- Divide trainees into pairs.
- Randomly assign a child to a pair of observers who will observe the same child in the classroom and in the playground. The same procedure will be carried out for the rest of the observer pairs.
- Ask trainees to focus on the level of gross and fine motor activities of the selected child, and note down all the relevant observations, especially focusing on the context of the observations.
- Make sure that the time duration for the observation in both settings is same, in order to have a standardized procedure.

Questions for discussion:
The facilitator can generate discussion on the experience that each pair had during observation.
- He or she can talk about the difference they find between observation in the classroom and in the playground i.e. about the level of gross and fine motor skills that can be changed due to change of context.
- He or she can ask which setting they find easier to observe and where they faced challenges.
- The facilitator can encourage the participants to reflect on what their usual routine way of observation is, and how these differ from the standardized observation.

Learning outcome:
- This activity will provide an opportunity to the participants to understand the importance of context for any observation.
- It will enable them to understand that change in the setting could change the behaviour pattern of a child.

Activity 2: *Role Play*

Title: Practices of reward and punishment

Goal: To develop the ability to observe child rearing practices.

VARIATIONS
- *Settings for observation can be different, the home, day care centre, or any playground near the home etc. where the child can be observed.*
- *Various child behaviours can be observed, such as cognitive functioning and interpersonal relationship with parents or peers etc.*

Objectives:

To identify the childrearing practices related to:

- Punishment
- Reward

Duration: 2 hours

Trainer Preparation:

- Note pad, pencil and eraser.
- Conduct role play preferably in a closed space, as some participants may not feel comfortable performing their roles in an open space.

Method:

- Divide participants into two groups, and assign each group a scenario to act on.
- For one group, the role-play scenario would be "where a child is rewarded on getting a good grade in the school exam" while the other group can be asked to act on the scene "where a child is being punished because of not getting a good grade in school exams".
- Provide a checklist to the rest of the participants to record the observations of the role-play. (See Appendix).
- After the role-play, ask every participant about his or her observation about the given items in the checklist.

Questions for discussion:

- At the end of collecting observations about the role-play from all the participants, the facilitator can highlight whether the observations have been comprehensively recorded or not.
- He/she can even ask if anything which emerged from the role play can be added, which is not currently the part of the checklist.
- Participants can be encouraged to point out, from their daily life experiences, other punishment and reward practices that prevail around them.

Learning outcome:

- This activity will provide an opportunity to the participants to understand and experience conventional roles, responsibilities and expectations of different types of caregivers.
- It will help them to focus their attention objectively on observation of the behaviours and events.

VARIATION

Role play of different type of care givers such as mother, father, sibling, relatives and child care service providers e.g. health educators etc. can be done.

Activity 3: *Field Visit*

Title: Age appropriate play of children

Goal: To develop skills of observing various types of children's play.

Objectives:

To observe various types of age appropriate play;

- Sensory motor play
- Constructive play
- Pretend play
- Substitute pretend play
- Socio dramatic play

Duration: 4 hours

Trainer Preparation:

- Note pad, pencil and eraser.
- Preliminary arrangement of logistics, for instance, venue (day care centre), transport, advance information to the administration of the day care centre.

Method:

- Visit a day care centre to observe children aged between 0 to 3 years.
- Divide trainees into 5 groups.
- Randomly assign a child to each group and ask them to observe the child at playtime.
- Ask them to focus on the types of the play of the selected child and note down all the relevant observations.
- Make sure that the time duration for the observation is an hour for all the observers to have standardized procedure.

Questions for discussion:

- The facilitator can generate a discussion about the experience of each group during observation:
- By taking their views regarding the contents of play changes with age, the importance of different types of play at different ages can be highlighted, while relating it with observations from participants.
- They need to be encouraged to share the joys and problems they may have encountered during the observation.
- Look for opportunities for children to explore the world through age appropriate play in their neighbourhoods and families.

Learning outcome:

- This activity will provide an opportunity to participants to have an in depth understanding of the child's play.
- They will be able to comprehend the importance of opportunities of holistic child development for age appropriate play in development.

Supportive considerations
Challenges during scientific observations

For scientific observation, it is always best to use a pre-tested and valid checklist.

- Sometimes observers forget to note information on the checklist; later this can create ambiguity, making it difficult to decide about whether the event took place or not, and whether they missed it or the event did not actually happen. To avoid this sort of ambiguity, it is recommended that the checklist be completed before leaving the place of observation.

- Children and caregiver behave differently when they feel the presence of the stranger who is observing them. This problem can be solved by not letting them know that they are under observation. However, this might lead to certain ethical issues. Another way of dealing with this is to build rapport with the child and the caregiver so that the threat of being observed will be lessened gradually and they will come to behave normally in the presence of the observer.

- Scientific observations should minimize biases, but this is not always easy. The observer has some views about what behaviour should be expected in a particular situation, which may be due to knowledge of the results of past investigations, or by the observer's own hypothesis about behaviour in the situation. Sometimes, this bias can be controlled by limiting the knowledge of the observer

> **VARIATION**
> *Settings for the observation can be different: at home, or in any playground near the home etc, where the child can be observed.*

chapter seven

QUESTIONNAIRE-BASED INTERVIEWS

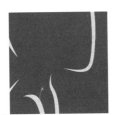

Learning Objectives

By the end of the session, participants would be able to:

- Define the term 'interview'.

- Recognize different types of questions used in interviews.

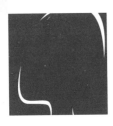

- Identify advantages and disadvantages of different types of questions.

- Identify different portions of a questionnaire and their importance.

- Delineate the steps involved in mapping and sampling in the field, and recruit eligible respondents who are caregivers of children.

- Identify the need for pre-testing of a questionnaire.

- Recognize the importance of informed consent.

- Identify issues related to refusals of interviews and their remedies. Enlist the measures required to maintain the quality of data.

Activity 1: Brainstorming

Title: Reward and punishment to the child

Goal: To develop mechanism to generate information for Early Childhood Development related themes.

Objectives:
To identify and discuss the themes of reward and punishment for 0-6 year old children from the perspective of caregivers specifically for:

- Situations of reward and punishment
- Reasons of reward and punishment
- Applied methods of reward and punishment

Duration: 2 hours

Trainer Preparation:
- Flipcharts and markers.
- Enough space for seating small groups, so that any one group's working remains undisturbed by adjacent groups' discussions.

Method:
- Divide the participants into two groups.
- Distribute markers & flipcharts to each group.
- Brief them, so that one group will take the topic of reward and the second group will take punishment part.
- Ask each group to come with thoughts and comments regarding situations when reward or punishment is given to a child, the reasons for reward and punishment and the methods adopted for each in their community.
- This task should be achieved through group discussion in a given time of 45 minutes.
- In the end both the groups sum up their discussion and share it with each other and with the facilitator.

Questions for discussion:
- The facilitator can generate discussion one by one on each segment like situation, reason and methods of rewards and punishment given to the child.
- The facilitator can encourage the participants to share their views that on how these practices of reward and punishment could affect child development.
- Participants encouraged to share the disciplinary practices they generally use for children and reflect on how such practices could affect the child's personality.

Learning outcome:
- This activity will enable them to generate themes related to early childhood development.
- It could be a helpful source for bringing awareness about the prevailing child caring practices and their consequences.

Activity 2: *Field Visit*

Title: Mapping and framework

VARIATIONS

- *The same activity could be done with various themes such as quality time given by caregivers, effects of pre-lacteal feed etc.*
- *This activity can be conducted from the perspective of fathers, mothers, grandparents, health service provider etc.*

Goal: To identify children in the community.

Objective:
To identify eligible children for the ECD community based development and research-related projects.

Duration: 4 hours

Trainer Preparation:
- Note pad, pencils and erasers.
- Chalk.
- Recording performa.
- Arrangement of logistics before time, for instance, venue (locality), transport, advance information to the concerned people.

Method:
- Begin by dividing participants into 5 groups.
- Distribute chalk, pencils, erasers and recording performa.
- Ask them to map 5 streets of a locality, by enquiring if children of 0-6 years of age are present in those houses. Allocate identification numbers on the door/wall of those houses where eligible children of the respective community are residing.
- Also record the age and sex of the child and the house identification number on the recording performa.
- Ask the participants to finish this activity of mapping within one hour.
- The facilitator should randomly check to see how the participants are working at their activity.
- Once all participants have completed their tasks, check the proformas and inquire about any difficulty in performing the activity.

Questions for discussion:
- The facilitator can ask the participants about the concept of mapping and its utility with respect to community development and research related projects.
- Encourage them to share the issues and challenges faced during the process of mapping.

Learning outcome:
- This activity will enable the participants to develop the skill of mapping according to the need of the project, to identify the eligible persons.
- The participants will learn to organize the information in a systematic fashion, by forming the framework to include all the identified eligible children.

Activity 3: *Role-play and Field activity*

Title: Interviewing techniques

Goal: To collect information about child rearing practices from caregivers.

Objective:
To conduct interview with caregiver on reward and punishment practices, while considering at least these issues:

VARIATION
Different study populations can be considered, e.g., pregnant women or children between the ages of 1 to 3 years.

- Informed consent
- Handling of refusal
- Sensitivity of information
- Confidentiality

Duration: 4 hours

Trainer Preparation:
- A questionnaire having set of questions related to reward and punishment practices. (see appendix for a sample).
- Note pad, pencil and eraser.
- Preliminary arrangement of logistics, for instance, venue, transport, advance information to the concerned people. Keep in mind the cultural sensitivity of that locality.

Method:
- Ask any two participants to volunteer to role-play as mother and interviewer.
- Ask the interviewer to highlight during role-play, the issues of informed consent, handling of refusal, sensitivity of information and confidentiality.
- Ask the rest of the participants to observe them, and at the end of role-play ask all participants to tell one by one what was actually going on in the play and how both characters in the role play reacted to that situation.
- Then take the participants to the community and ask them to visit the homes of the eligible children and fill out at least 2 forms individually.
- Ask them to note down how they handled the given issues.

Questions for discussion:
- The facilitator can ask them to share their field experience.
- Generate discussion about the importance of informed consent, issue of confidentiality, sensitivity of information obtained, and handling of refusal, by keeping in mind all the responses given by the participants.
- Ask them to reflect on what they felt when they had hands-on experience in the field, and encourage them to share their apprehensions and challenges in performing such activity in the future.

Learning outcomes:
- This activity will enable participants to practice informed consent, issue of confidentiality, sensitivity of information and handling of refusal during field activities.
- This activity will help them to identify actively the issues and prospects of better child development at the community level.

VARIATIONS
- *The topic of the question can be changed, e.g., the practice of giving pre-lacteal feed, quality time, hygiene and sanitation etc.*
- *Same activity could be done with other caregivers like father and grandparents.*

chapter eight

FOCUS GROUP DISCUSSION

Learning Objectives

By the end of the session, participants would be able to:

- Define the term "Focus Group Discussion" (FGD).

- Differentiate focus group from general discussion and group interview.

- List different steps for the preparation of a Focus Group Discussion.

- Define the general process of conducting a Focus Group Discussion.

- List types of focus group discussions.

- Describe positive experience of child development at community level.

- Define the concept of positive deviance for ECD.

- Describe a conceptual framework of conducting a positive deviance inquiry.

- Identify the utility of conducting Focus Group Discussions in relation to Early Childhood Development.

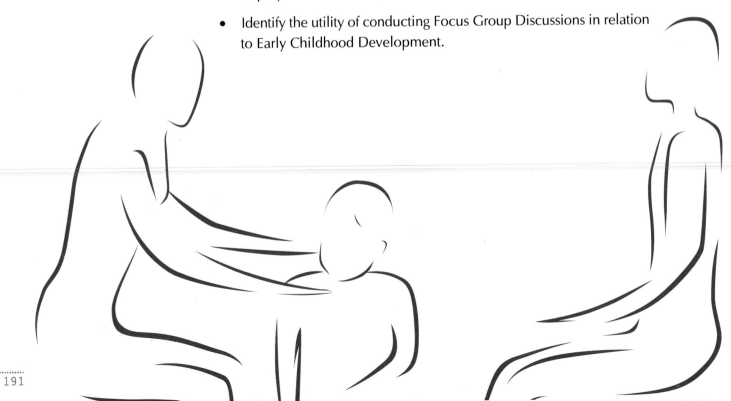

Activity 1: *Group Discussion*

Title: Understanding of focus group discussion

Goal: To develop an understanding of focus group discussion as a planned activity.

Objective:
To identify and discuss different steps of preparation of focus group discussion.

Duration: 2 hours

Trainer Preparation:
- Small colourful cards on which different focus group preparation-related terms are written, like target group, time duration, group size, composition of group, discussion guidelines, tape recorder etc.

Method:
- Place all the written cards face down on the floor or table.
- Ask one by one all participants to pick one card randomly, (so that they cannot see what topic they choose).
- Make them all sit in a large circle and ask them one by one to talk about his or her topic to the rest of the participants; they should explain to others their own understanding of that term. For instance, a participant may get a card of time duration, in which case he or she tells other participants about the meaning of time duration in focus group discussion.

Questions for discussion:
- At the end of the explanation of each topic by the participants, the facilitator can generate discussion on the need and importance of that topic for the focus group discussion.
- Ask particpants to express their views about the consequences of inadequate preparation for focus group discussion during the discussion session.
- The facilitator should sum up the discussion by enhancing the importance of an ideal situation for the FGD.

Learning outcome:
- This activity will enable them to have a clear understanding of the need for preparation of FGD.
- It will enable them to learn about skills related to logistical support, an important prerequisite for the successful conduct of focus group discussion.

Activity 2: *Group Activity*

Title: Interviewing techniques

Goal: To develop an understanding of focus group discussion and the skills related to conduct of focus group discussion.

Objectives:
- To develop discussion guidelines for the FGD at least on:
  - □ Prelacteal feed given to the child at the time of birth
  - □ Role of fathers in childcare
- To understand and practice the roles of key persons of FGD

VARIATIONS
- *These topic, related to preparation for focus group discussion can be further divided in their sub-domains: for example, the target group in a focus group discussion can be considered on the basis of sex, socio-economic status etc.*
- *The same activity could be done for the understanding of roles and responsibilities of the facilitator, observer and note taker.*

Duration: 4 hours

Trainer Preparation:
- Note pads, pencil and eraser.

Method:
- Divide the participants into two groups. One group is given the topic about prelacteal feed while the other one is given the role of the father in childcare.
- Ask each group to write down the possible questions related to the topic i.e. the discussion guideline, which they could use to get information on their topic from a focus group discussion. (30 min); they should not share these guidelines with the other group's members.
- Ask each group for volunteers to take on the role of facilitator, observer and note-taker, and to conduct the FGD for about an hour with the rest of the participants.
- The same process needs to be carried out for the second group.

Questions for discussion:
- The facilitator can ask questions on the discussion guidelines, and can generate discussion on the relevance of the discussion guidelines and their importance to the theme to be explored.
- The facilitator can help the participants to highlight the role played by the players.
- In a focus group discussion, the facilitator encourages member of the group to share their learning and apprehensions with him/her and other participants.

VARIATION

Discussion guidelines can be generated on various themes, such as the role of caregivers and health service providers, and the importance of stimulating environment for the child, etc.

Learning outcome:
- This activity will enable participants to learn the skill of preparing discussion guidelines, and understanding the roles of different key people for the focus group discussions.
- The process will help participants learn the skills of recording discussion information, and understand group dynamics, and learn ways of probing and facilitation.

Activity 3: *Field Visit*
Title: Positive Deviance

Goal: To create an understanding and importance of positive deviance.

Objective:
To conduct a focus group discussion related to positive deviance with a group of teachers, who teach children of the same class level.

Duration: 4 hours

Trainer Preparation:
- Focus group discussion guidelines that must be developed after considering cultural sensitivities.
- Note pads, pencil and eraser.
- Preliminary arrangement of logistics, for instance, venue (day care centre), visit timing, transport, advance information to the concerned people.

Method:
- Make a group comprising 3 participants in which one a facilitator and the remaining two are observer and note taker.
- Begin the discussion by asking the teachers to share their positive experiences related to students'

achievement.

- During that discussion, identify those teachers who may have remarkable achievements in making their class or student progress well.
- Probe them about the efforts they took to achieve such success
- Ask the rest of the participants what they can do to better their situations while being in the same environment.
- Continue discussion for a maximum of one and a half hours.

Questions for discussion:

- The facilitator inquires about the responses given by the FGD's participants and can relate them with the concept of positive deviance.
- Ask all the participants to give their view about the importance of highlighting the positive deviants for community development.
- Encourage participants to reflect on whatever they have learnt from this activity and share their concerns regarding conduct of such activity independently in the future.

Learning outcome:

- This activity will enable participants to learn skills of conducting focus group discussions in real settings.
- It will help participants to see the effectiveness of experiential learning, and will enable them to analyse the importance of positive deviants in a community.

Supportive considerations

Logistics & Setup

- For time allocation, consider the convenience of the participants regarding the time they can easily manage for focus group discussion. It is also necessary to inform participants about the period in advance, and to honor the agreed time limit.

Physical Environment

- The first step is to identify a place, which is accessible for participants to come to. It is important to try and identify a place, which is large enough to accommodate the group, and is well lit.

- Take into account the need and convenience of participants for the preference of seating arrangements. It is preferable to make the participants sit in a circle, so that each participant can see the other participants and the facilitator. In urban areas it is better to have a comfortable round table seating arrangement while in rural areas, floor seating might be more appropriate, being in line with cultural traditions.

Record

- In recording a FGD using a tape recorder, one has to acknowledge the noise factor in the environment that usually affects the quality of recording; perhaps in such circumstances a note taker might be a better option in addition to tape recording. If the FGD is to be tape-recorded, the preliminary checking for availability of the equipment and testing is highly recommended.

- A translator is required when the researchers do not speak the local language. In this case, a translator needs to be identified and orientated prior to the FGD, and allowances should be made for the possibility of more time needed to conduct the FGD, especially for understanding of responses and questions.

VARIATION

This activity can be conducted with various groups of caregivers like elder siblings, grandparents, and parents of children of the same age. This can also work well with health and/or education service providers working on the same area of childcare.

chapter nine

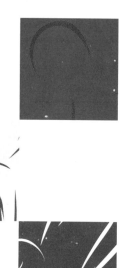

COMMUNICATION SKILLS

Learning Objectives

By the end of the session, participants would be able to:

- Define communication.

- Describe conceptual model of communication.

- Discuss factors enabling effective communication.

- Classify types of communication.

- Define domains of human communication.

- Describe the cautions required while communicating with different ECD groups.

- Describe role of interviewer as a speaker as well as a listener.

- Define counselling.

- Classify type of counselling encountered by ECD workers.

- Describe process of counselling.

- Enlist verbal and non-verbal counselling skills.

- Delineate use of counselling in relation to communication skills in ECD.

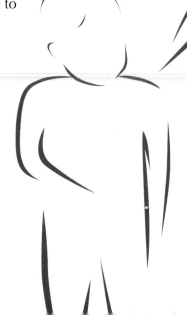

Activity 1: *Brainstorming*

Title: Role of communication skills in child rearing practices

Goal: To develop an understanding of how to communicate effectively.

Objective:
To identify factors enabling effective communication to the caregiver of young children by focusing on: sender 'message', receiver 'feedback'.

Duration: 2 hours

Trainer Preparation:
- Flipcharts and markers.
- Enough space for seating small groups, so that any one group's working remains undisturbed by adjacent groups' discussions.

Method:
- Divide the participants into small groups of five members each.
- Distribute Markers & Flipcharts to each group.
- Brief them to give comments regarding how to communicate proper hand washing practices to the caregivers in their own community.
- Advise them to keep in mind the basic components of communication including sender, message, receiver and feedback.
- This task should be achieved through group discussion in a given time of 45 minutes.
- Now ask each group to present their discussion.

Questions for discussion:
- Ask participants' opinion on the barriers to communicating health related messages at the household level, and ask for their suggestions on overcoming these hurdles.

Learning outcome:
- This activity will help participants to develop the skills of a good communicator. They will be able to identify the barriers to good communication, which are important for the caregiver for child development related messages within their own context.

> **VARIATION**
> **This exercise can also be done by social workers, by changing the topic to communication of antenatal care related messages for pregnant women.**

Activity 2: *Group Work*

Title: A Quad of listeners

Goal: To illustrate the importance of careful listening

Objective:
To make participants understand the importance of understanding by listening to other peoples' communication with them.

Duration: 2 hours

Trainer Preparation:

- Note pads, pencils and erasers.
- Preferably in a closed space, as some participants may not feel comfortable performing their ro[le]
  in an open space.

Method:

- Begin by dividing participants into four groups.
- Assign for identification, letters of the alphabet to each group e.g., "T", "A", "L", "K" to all f[our]
  groups.
- Assign one critical element of the social environment to each of the following groups
    - Group "T" – Internal relationships
    - Group "A" – External relationships
    - Group "L" – External services
    - Group "K" – Socio-cultural & Political context
- Ask each group to converse about the ways in which they can improve in the context of early ch[ild]
  development one by one.
- Advise the participants to listen carefully.
- Group "T" will start the talk. After that, ask group "A" to paraphrase in their own words what th[ey]
  have understood from the talk of group "T". After that, group "A" will speak on their assigned top[ic]
  and group "L" will paraphrase. When group "L" speaks, group "T" will paraphrase.
- The remaining participants will be required to listen carefully. Jot down the barriers to listenin[g]
  experienced during the talk of each group.
- Ask each group to summarize their observations and make separate presentations.

Questions for discussion:

- The facilitator can discuss different factors required to be an effective listener, and the barriers th[ey]
  encounter during listening.

VARIATION

The topic for discussion can be changed to child rearing practices in the context of early child development.

Learning outcome:

- The participants will develop an understanding of the fact that an important aspect of effecti[ve]
  communication is effective listening. They will learn the skill and significance of effective listenin[g.]

Activity 3: *Role Play*

Title: Gender differentials in child rearing practices

Goal: To develop the skills required to counsel caregivers of young children.

Objectives:
To develop an understanding of counselling in terms of:
- Process
- Types
- Skills

Duration: 2 hours

Trainer Preparation:
- Preferably in a closed space, as some participants may not feel comfortable performing their rol[e]
  in an open space.

Method:

- Brief them on how to nominate two members from their particular group to play the assigned role.
- Ask participants for two volunteers for role-playing of this activity: of the volunteers, one would play the role of primary care giver (mother/father) of 3-year-old twin children, a boy and the girl. The second participant would assume the role of a social worker.
- Brief them to start the discussion at the point where both the twin children are playing with a bat and a ball. However, the care provider asks the girl to stop playing with her brother, and instead play with her doll. The worker should start the talk by asking the caregiver for the reasons for the exclusion of the girl from the game that both children were playing. The caregiver refuses to answer, as she/he considers that she/he was acting according to the age old customs prevalent in her area.
- After some resistance, the worker succeeds in persuading her to discuss the issue. During the discussion, the worker explains to the caregiver that both girls and boys are equal, and counsels them not to deprive the girl from a game of bat and ball, just she because is a girl. The worker faces lot of questions, but she tackles them tactfully, by using her interviewing and counseling skills.
- Ask the remaining participants to observe the role play, and focus on the process of counselling.

Questions for discussion:

- At the end of the roleplay obtain feedback from the remaining participants regarding the whole process of counselling. Ask them whether the worker has properly carried out the process of counselling; also ask, which types of counselling she had utilized, and which of the verbal and non verbal clues they have identified from the process.

Learning outcome:

- This activity will help participants develop counseling skills, and overcome hindrances faced during the process.
- Participants will also learn persuasion techniques for desired practices, and ways of expressing disapproval of undesired practices in an effective manner.

VARIATION

Individuals can be asked to do the same activity with a teacher or a community leader of their area.

chapter ten

COMMUNITY DYNAMICS

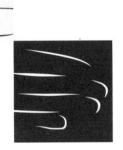

Learning Objectives

By the end of the session, participants would be able to:

- Define the term 'Community' in the context of early childhood development.

- Differentiate between rural and urban communities.

- List the general attributes that contribute to the composition of communities.

- Express a basic understanding of the importance of the community in early childhood development programs.

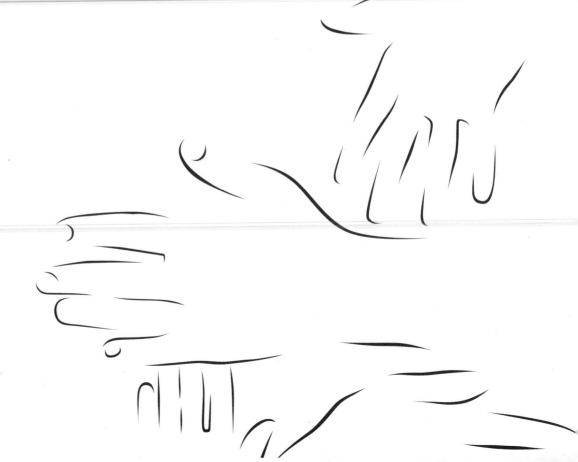

Activity 1: *Field Visit*

Title: Community Dynamics

Goal: To develop an understanding of the distinguishing features of different types of communities in the context of ECD.

Objectives:
- To appreciate the difference between urban and rural communities in relation to living style, source of income, education and cultural traditions
- To develop an understanding of critical elements of the social environment, as applied in community settings
- o Internal relationships
- o External relationships
- o External services
- o Socio-cultural and Political context

Duration: 4 hours

Trainer Preparation:
- Have information on cultural norms readily available.
- Note pad, pencils and erasers.
- Preliminary arrangement of logistics, for instance, venue (school, household), visit timing, transport, advance information to the concerned people

Method:
- Divide participants into two groups.
- Have one group visit an urban site and the other a rural site.
- Prepare a field visit guide to explain the method of collecting information through observations and a simple interview on living style, source of income, education and cultural traditions in relation to:
  - □ Internal relationships
  - □ External relationships
  - □ External services
  - □ Socio-cultural and Political context
- Participants can be asked to make brief 10 minutes presentations summarizing their visits.

Questions for discussion:
- The facilitator can ask participants to compare the difference in features observed during their visit to specific sites. Differences can be noted in living style, source of income, education and cultural traditions among the two community settings. Ask questions about the extent of existing resources such as education or health care. Participants can also reflect upon the deciding factors for selection of a community for initiating an ECD programme.

Learning outcome:
- Participants will learn the skill of interaction with a community and gain community orientation.
- Participants will go through the process of reaching a final decision on selection of communities

VARIATION
Observations about community dynamics among different ethnic groups of community dynamics.

Supportive considerations

Some important points to make the ECD Programes more successful in communities

Here is a review of some of the important points before starting any programme related to Early Childhood Development in a community:

- Information about the community can be collected through reports and maps, or from any organization working in the area, and through interviews with informants such as health workers or leaders.

- Establishing contact with and selection of community leaders.

- Selection of time and venue convenient to community members (adopt a flexible approach) before conducting a meeting.

- Introduction of the study, its goals and objectives to community leaders (zamindar, wadera, counsellor, elected or appointed officers, etc.)

- Learning to respect the cultural norms and other values of the community.

- Laying emphasis on meaningful community participation.

- Involving community volunteers.

- Identifying paid workers in the absence of volunteers.

- Making Terms of Reference (TOR) for paid workers.

chapter eleven

ECD PROGRAM DEVELOPMENT

Learning Objectives

By the end of the session, participants would be able to:

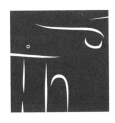

- Describe a community based ECD program.

- Identify stages of a planning cycle.

- Describe steps of situation analysis for a communitybased ECD program.

- Outline the process of priority setting.

- List the criteria for developing objectives.

- Describe the mechanism of transforming objectives into program activities.

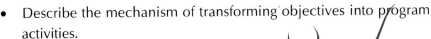

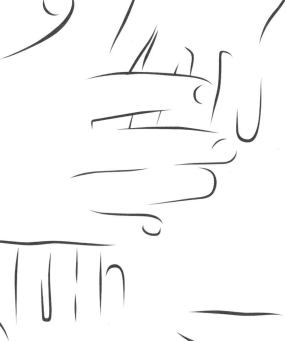

Activity 1: *Group activity*

Title: Sources for needs assessment

Goal: To develop understanding of different sources of information for ECD indicators.

Objectives:
To identify the sources of information for ECD indicators through specified methodologies.
- Observations
- Surveys
- Documents

Duration: 2 hours

Trainer Preparation:
- Note pad, pencils and erasers
- Exercise working material (e.g. attached).

Method:
- Distribute exercise-working material (note pad, pencils and table of ECD indicators) among the participants.
- Give instructions to participants on the ways in which data on each indicator can be collected from the possible given sources of information.
- Inform participants about the time required to complete the exercise (20 minutes).
- For each indicator there can be more than one methodology.

Questions for discussion:
- Generate discussion on the pros and cons of different sources of information for ECD indicators.
- Ask the participants about the utility of this information in situation analysis, especially needs assessment and priority setting.
- Think about why some sources are more comfortable to work with as compared to others, and the reasons for those differences.

Learning outcome:
- Participants will develop the skill of identification of various sources of information for ECD indicators, and learn the importance of assessment of ECD indicators in the context of situation analysis
- Participants will be able to appreciate the importance of different sources of information for ECD indicators through specified methodologies such as observations, surveys and documents

VARIATION
Data collection methodologies can be suggested, and participants can be asked to suggest relevant ECD indicators, which can be easily assessed by specific methodology.

Assessing Needs	Information sources		
Questions	Visits	Surveys	Documents
A. Internal relationships: child's interaction within a family			
1) Do parents give quality time to children?			
2) Are all components of nutrients available in the home daily diet?			
3) Is learning material provided to the child?			
4) Are sewage lines in the house and community covered?			
5) Are rotary electrical fans covered?			
6) Is access to stairs restricted for younger children?			
B. External relationships: interaction in neighborhood, school and playgrounds			
1) Coverage of children according to age specific vaccination schedule for children <5			
2) Antenatal care received through trained health professionals			
3) Proportion of eligible children attending primary schools			
4) Average number of visits to health care facility annually by children <5			
5) Average amount of time child spends playing at the playground daily			
C. External services: work place and community health services			
Structure of health facilities: doctors, nurses and dispensaries available			
1) Number of schools in the community and up to what level			
2) Availability of safe drinking water			
3) Number of playgrounds in the community			
D. Child growth and developmental status			
1) Proportion of children regularly monitored for height and weight			
2) Proportion of children weighing less than 2500 grams at birth			
3) Can the child take part in activities like running or jumping			
4) Can the child stack small blocks			
5) Is the child able to solve puzzles			
6) Involvement in playing hide and seek games			
7) Child's ability to recognize pictures, printed letters or words and matching sounds			
8) Whether child is happy on seeing parents, siblings			
9) Can the child understand language			
10) Can the child communicate thoughts verbally			
E. Sociocultural and political context			
1) Primary schools for girls			
2) Implementation of child labor laws in the community			
3) Predominant family type (Joint or nuclear family system)			
F. Significant life events			
1) Admission to a school			
2) Children repeating classes			
3) Drop-outs from schools			
4) Death of immediate family member / birth of siblings			
5) Natural calamities in the community (e.g. flood, storm etc)			

Activity 2: *Field activity*

Title:
Social services for ECD

Goal: To develop an understanding of social services and their integration to create a conducive environment for children at community level.

Objectives:
- To identify social services involved in ECD such as:
  - Health care
  - Education
  - Public works
- To understand issues and challenges in integration of these social services

Duration: 4 hours

Trainer Preparation:
- Note pad, pencils and erasers.
- Arrangement of logistics before time, for instance, venue (school, household), visit timing, transport, advance information to the concerned people.

Method:
- Divide participants into two groups.
- Brief the team on the purpose of the visit, and give instructions on collection of information about extent of services available in the community, according to a list of respective services.
- The first group can collect information on education services.
- The second group can collect information on health care services.
- Ask the groups to visit community leaders and specific service organizations, to inquire about the relevant information that they need.
- The groups will present their findings regarding issues and challenges concerning the integration of services in the community.

> **VARIATION**
> *Structure of social services in urban and rural communities can be compared.*

Questions for discussion:
- The facilitator can ask participants about the types of services available, and
- The existing level of cooperation among social services in the community.
- The facilitator can ask for the reasons for lack of communication and cooperation among social service providers to achieve their common goal of child development.
- Participants can reflect on ways in which the situation can be improved.

Learning outcome:
- Development of skills of communication with relevant social services.
- Development of understanding of the strengths and weaknesses of these social services.
- Conceptualization of strategies to integrate these social services.

Activity 3: *Group activity*

Title: Planning cycle for ECD programmes

Goal: To develop an understanding of the planning cycle for ECD programs.

Objectives:
- To identify the steps involved in preparation of the planning cycle of ECD programs.
- To plan an ECD program by focusing on the critical elements of the social environment.
  - ☐ Internal relationships
  - ☐ External relationships
  - ☐ External services
  - ☐ Socio-cultural and Political context

Duration: 2 hours

Trainer Preparation:
- Note pads, pencils and erasers.

Method:
- Divide participants into two groups.
- Brief the groups about the method of activities to be undertaken, e.g., the participants will be required to sit down and start discussion in their respective groups.
- Each group can select their own moderator for discussion.
- Ask the first group to plan a strategy for children's hygiene, while the second group does the same for immunization status of children.
- The task will be to begin with situation analysis, go on to priority setting, followed by programme implementation and evaluation for both strategies.
- At the end the groups will present a summary of their discussions in front of the whole team, in 10 minutes.

Questions for discussion:
- The facilitator can ask the groups to discuss how children's hygiene can be assessed within the community.
- The facilitator can ask about the planning which will be required to improve at the level of family hygiene, neighbourhood and schools, health care services and the community.
- Similarly, questions can also be asked on assessment of immunization status of children within a community.
- The facilitator can inquire about steps to be undertaken to improve immunization status of children by facilitating integration between stakeholders in a community.
- Participants can reflect on the practicality of the planned activities, and learn about ensuring sustainability of these activities.

VARIATION
Strategies can be planned for education and nutritional status of children.

Learning outcome:
- Participants will learn how to plan an ECD programe with specific objectives.
- Participants will develop an understanding of application of ECD programe planning according to the critical elements of the social environment.
  - ☐ Internal relationships
  - ☐ External relationships
  - ☐ External services
  - ☐ Socio-cultural and Political context

Supportive considerations

Participants will be given a short overview of this module in a classroom setting. Different components of the ECD program development would be discussed, with emphasis on implementation in the community.

In designing an ECD program, the following points should be kept in mind by the trainer:

- Program design allows innovations and flexibility at any stage, provided that they do not fall out from the main objectives. However, new objectives can be developed as part of this exercise, since this is a learning exercise for all.

- Shortcomings of the program design can be identified. Corrective action based on the learning experience of the participants must be recognized.

- While the team carries responsibility for the overall development of different tasks in the programme development, the trainer should emphasize the promotion of a culture of teamwork, and should be a source of motivation.

- It is emphasized that the participants should be properly recognized for their contribution.

chapter twelve

ECD PROGRAM MANAGEMENT

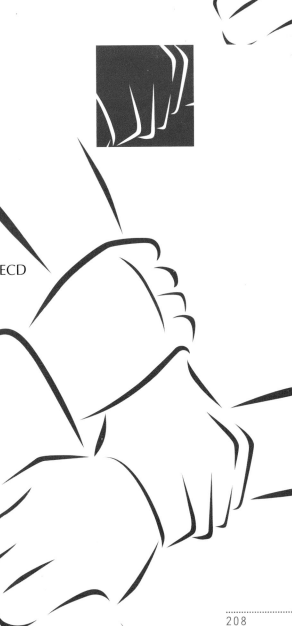

Learning Objectives

By the end of the session, participants would be able to:

- Describe the concept of Program Management.

- List the characteristics of a field coordinator.

- Identify mechanisms to form a community ECD committee.

- Describe the process of ECD field team development.

- Identify mechanisms to achieve timelines for the program.

- Generate a list of activities to develop capacity building of an ECD field team.

- List the elements of report writing.

- Identify ethical concerns in ECD programs.

Activity 1: *Brainstorming*

Title: Selection of community-based ECD committee

Goal: To understand and develop a formal mechanism of community participation for ECD initiatives.

Objectives:
To identify steps in the formation of:
- A community-based ECD committee.
- Development of TOR for the ECD committee in consultation with the community.

Duration: 2 hours

Trainer Preparation:
- Note pads, pencils and erasers.

Method:
- The facilitator can ask the participants to sit in a circle.
- The facilitator can distribute pencils and paper to all participants.
- Ask them to write down their characteristics i.e., strengths, individual skills and motivation for being involved in ECD programming.
- The facilitator should ask the group to share these characteristics and select members for a community based ECD committee, on the basis of their merit.
- The group will then decide about selection of the most adequate representatives from the community to be included in the community ECD committee.
- The facilitator will ask the participants to develop TORs for the formation of a community ECD committee. Some of the important considerations for the TORs are:
  - Objectives
  - Identification of stakeholders
  - Representation
  - Discipline
  - Schedule for meetings
  - Venue
  - Timeframe
  - Quorum
- TORs should define roles and responsibilities of individual team members.

Questions for discussion:
- Ask the participants about how regular functioning of the committee can be ensured by committee members.
- Ask participants to discuss the individual level skills that members should bring to the committee.
- The facilitator should encourage discussion on responsibilities of individual committee members.
- Participants can also reflect on the contributions they can make in such committees.

Learning outcome:
- Participants learn skills for selection of the right people for a community ECD committee.
- Participants can develop skills for improving community participation.
- Development of criteria for TORs of a community ECD based committee.

VARIATION

In a conservative cultural setup a 'women's only' community-based committee for ECD can be formed.

Activity 2: *Group Activity*

VARIATION
Distribution of cards with a list of responsibilities: participants will allocate appropriate roles for specific responsibilities .

Title: Responsibilities of stakeholders in community-based ECD programmes.

Goal: To understand that ECD stakeholders have defined roles and responsibilities in the social environment of a child.

Objectives:
To list individual roles and responsibilities of different ECD stakeholders such as:

- Coordinator
- Supervisor
- ECD committee member
- ECD community worker
- Caregiver
- Community leader
- Religious leader
- Representative of the government
- Health care service provider

Duration: 2 hours

Trainer Preparation:
- Small cards.
- Note pads, pencils and erasers.

Method:
- The facilitator should distribute cards with the names of stakeholders written on them.
- Participants should then make a list of responsibilities for each stakeholder.
- Participants should be asked to present responsibilities of stakeholders in brief 5-minute presentations.
- Each participant can have a turn at presenting responsibilities.

Questions for discussion:
- The facilitator can ask participants about childcare responsibilities which can be shared by multiple stakeholders, despite their specific roles. Participants can reflect on roles and responsibilities as caregivers in their own community setups. For example, feeding a child can be done by different people, and it will be clear after the exercise that this can be taken up by any assigned person if the mother/father is unable to feed the child.

Learning outcome:
- Participants will develop skills to identify particular sets of responsibilities for different roles of stakeholders in the social environment of children.
- Participants will develop the understanding that ECD requires an integrated approach, by sharing of responsibilities and roles.

Activity 3: *Role Playing*

Title: Ethical Issues in ECD

Goal: To develop the basic understanding of ethical principles in the context of ECD programmes

Respect

Beneficence

Justice

Objectives:

To identify ethical considerations pertinent to critical elements of the social environment for ECD.

- Internal relationships
- External relationships
- External services
- Socio-cultural and Political context

Duration: 2 hours

Trainer Preparation:

- Note pad, pencil and eraser.

Method:

- Divide participants into four groups.
- Brief them on how to nominate two members from their particular group to play the assigned roles. Role-playing should follow a consensus.
- Assign each group a critical element of the social environment, by playing out roles particular to that element in relation to ethical issues.
  - ☐ Group one – Internal relationships (Mother is feeding her children after they are back from school).
  - ☐ Group two – External relationships (e.g. Class visit to the national museum with schoolteachers).
  - ☐ Group three – External services (District health officer is explaining the importance of hygiene to children at the local BHU).
  - ☐ Group four – Socio-Cultural & Political context (Community ECD committee meeting to discuss availability of clean drinking water in the community).
- Each group will conduct the role play for 10 minutes.
- Ask role players to apply basic ethical principles in the context of the critical element of the social environment given to them.
- The remaining participants will make necessary observations, and note whether the principles of respect, beneficence and justice are being followed or not.
- Each group will summarize observations and make 10-minute presentations at the end.

Questions for discussion:

- Discuss each role play in the context of the ethical principles of:

Respect

Beneficence

Justice

- For reflection, the facilitator can ask members of each group about their response if they were to observe any breach of ethical principles in a community setting, and the possible solutions they would provide to the problem.

Learning outcome:

- Appreciation of child rights.

VARIATION

Participants can list different ethical issues arising in the household, health care setups, schools and community settings.

- Sensitization to the concept of ethics.
- Development of skills to identify vulnerable situations for children.
- Learning to respond to ethical issues as their social and moral responsibility.

Supportive considerations

Some important considerations for trainers:

- The facilitator should emphasize the importance of sustainability, which is only possible when community members own the program and provide sufficient support.

- To achieve sustainability, the importance of local capacity building should be highlighted, as this will ensure the availability of knowledgeable persons with reasonable skills to manage successfully the ECD programmes in the community.

- Record keeping is very important for measuring the success of the program, as well as for provision of audit for their resources and activities.

- Describe the importance of a flow chart to the participants.

- Give examples of experiences in community settings.

- Explain the importance of ethical concerns to the participants.

List of exercises in teaching and training section

Ch. #	Chapter Name	Brainstorming	Field Visit	Role Play	Group Activity
1	Fundamentals of Childhood Development	1	-	1	-
2	Social Environment	-	1	1	1
3	General Guidelines For Child Assessment	2	-	-	1
4	Nutrition, Growth and anthropometry	1	-	1	3
5	Intellectual Assessment	-	1	1	-
6	Observational Methodology	-	2	1	-
7	Questionnaire Based Interviews	1	1	1+FA*	-
8	Focus Group Discussions	-	1	1	1
9	Communication Skills	1	-	1	1
10	Community Dynamics	-	1	-	-
11	ECD Program Development	-	1	-	2
12	ECD Program Management	1	-	1	1

*FA Field Activity

Appendices

Developmental Milestones (1,2,3)

Developmental milestones observed could vary from child to child. In individual cases, children's milestones should not be referred to as delayed if the child does not perform the age-appropriate activities mentioned in this chart, until and unless confirmed by the clinician.

Age	Physical development	Cognitive Development	Socio-emotional Development
1 month	• Moves arms and legs vigorously. • Holds hands in fist most of the time	• More efficient in use of reflexes, can react differently to the pacifier and thumb. • Makes throaty noises. • Responds to primary caregiver's voice.	• Makes an eye contact with caregiver. • Shows distress by crying.
2 months	• Grasp reflex • Holds head upright most of the time when held in sitting position.	• Stops crying at the sight of mother's breast or bottle. • Follows moving objects.	• Social smile begins.
3 months	• Blinks to visual threat • While lying on one side turns from side to back. • Grasps an object voluntarily.	• Shows recognition memory; reacts to newness with body stiffening; grows quiet at the sight of an interesting toy. • Explores objects through touch. • Starts cooing.	• Excitement and boredom appear. • Matches adults' emotional expression during face to face interaction. • Turns head in the direction of familiar voice.
4months	• In prone position, lifts head and shoulders using arms.	• Anticipation becomes immediate; opens mouth at the sight of nipple. • Opens and closes hands. • Starts babbling.	• Laughs. • Shows beginnings of anger.
5 months	• While lying on back, can turn to the side. • Manipulates objects held in hands by rotating forearms.	• Imitates sound produced by the caregiver. • Observes any object held in hand.	• Some begin to show wariness of a stranger.
6 months	• While lying on back turns to prone position.	• Prefers brightly coloured objects. • Depth and pattern perception emerge and improve.	• Smiles and laughs when the caregiver does. • Recognizes and interacts with familiar persons other than primary caregiver.
7 months	• Supports his or her whole weight on legs. • Sits without support.	• Explores objects by manipulation. • Uses finger and thumb to grasp objects. • More attentive when playing. • Responds to his name.	• Reaches out when caregiver holds out her arms to the child.
8 months	• While lying on back, raises head and shoulders in an attempt to sit. • Transfers objects from one hand to the other.	• Repeats polysyllables. • Concentrates on one toy at a time.	• Touches and explores body parts. • Clings to the caregiver in the presence of a stranger.

Age	Physical development	Cognitive Development	Socio-emotional Development
9 months	• Starts crawling.	• Holds objects in each hand and brings them together.	• Recognizes self in mirror. • Shows negative emotion when restrained.
10 months	• Stands with support	• Explores inside and outside of the toy. • Repeats play sequence with different toys. • Starts to point with index finger • Speaks one word with meaning	• Prefers mother or regular care provider over all others. • Plays with the caregiver e.g. peek-a-boo.
11 months	• Walks sideways with support. • Uses pincer grasp.	• Uses props as aid e.g. uses a chair to stand up. • Comprehends simple words e.g. 'bye-bye'.	• Repeats sounds and gestures for attention. • Individual temperament is more evident. • Understands simple non-verbal communication by the caregiver's action and facial expression.
12 months	• Walks with one hand held. • Puts things into container.	• Searches for objects when they are hidden within sight. • Engages in intentional or goal directed behaviour. • Speaks at least three words with meaning.	• Becomes distressed when others are distressed. • Repeats acts that are praised by the caregiver.
15 months	• Walking is better coordinated. • Stands without support. • Can scribble.	• Recognizes and uses more cause and effect relationships. • Experiments with objects in a trial and error fashion. • Understands significance of "no".	• Shows signs of empathy. • Shows discomfort when familiar caregiver is out of sight.
18 months	• Builds towers of 2-3 cubes. • Walks without support.	• Has primitive ideas of "what should be" e.g., puts lids on jars. • Joins at least two words meaningfully to convey a thought. • Matches similar objects.	• Capable of compliance. • Can be restless and stubborn. • Imitates behaviour of others. • Considers his or her behaviour to be good.
21 months	• Walks confidently without tripping on obstacles. • Can pull and push objects.	• Identifies at least three objects at home. • Develops some understanding of categories e.g. colours.	• Refers to self as good or bad. • Begins to show defiant behaviour. • Begins to tolerate caregivers' absences more easily. • Begins to understand parent's values.
24 months	• Uses spoon effectively. • Runs with ease. • Assists while being dressed.	• Engages in make - believe play. • Refers to self both by noun and pronoun.	• Demonstrates increasing independence; expresses wide range of emotions. • Self control appears.

Age	Physical development	Cognitive Development	Socio-emotional Development
27 months	• Jumps forwards with both feet. • Holds pencil with thumb and fingers and draws on paper.	• Recognition memory well developed. • Follows directions involving preposition. • Understands the concept of "one".	• Understands causes and consequences of basic emotions (happiness, sadness, fear, anger etc). • Interacts with strangers even when familiar caregivers are not present.
30 months	• Walks in a straight line, heel touching toes. • Turns pages of a book one at a time	• Asks simple questions • Finds hidden objects of interest.	• Begins to show shame and embarrassment. • Expresses opinion about good or bad things.
33 months	• Walks on toes.	• Puts on and takes off clothes. • Differentiates between genders.	• Joint interplay increases.
36 months	• Stands on one foot.	• May be able to see the perspective of others. • Discriminates between colours.	• Assists in simple tasks. • Gender stereotyped beliefs and behaviour increases.
37 to 48 months	• Rides tricycle. • Jumping, hopping and throwing become better coordinated.	• Is able to understand the difference between parts of an object, and the whole. • Can generalize remembered information from one situation to another.	• Shows guilt and pride. • Instrumental aggression declines and hostile aggression increases.
49 to 60 months	• Large muscles skills increase in speed and endurance.	• Understands that letters and sounds are linked in a systematic way.	• Increase of understanding and use of emotional display rules. • Wants to please and be with friends. • More likely to agree to rules.
61 to 72 months	• Ties shoes, draws more elaborate pictures.	• Attention becomes more sustained and planned.	• Begins to understand how two or more emotions can occur simultaneously. • Ability to interpret, predict and influence others' emotional reactions improves. • Relies on language to express empathy. • Acquires many morally relevant rules and behaviour.

Weaning (Solid food introduction)

Before 6 months of age, there is no nutritional need for introducing solid foods. This is so because all the nutritional needs of an infant are fulfilled by breast milk, and they do not need any additional food, nor are they fully able to handle such foods. (4). By the age of 6 months most infants need food other than breast milk because they are physiologically and developmentally ready for it; there is also the need for iron.

- Weaning could be started by giving single foods initially, one at a time in small amounts.
- It is good to give a gap of 7 days between introducing each new food, in order to know whether the child is allergic to a particular food (5).

Guidelines For Food Introduction (6)

Age	Food	Type
0 -6 months	Breastfeed	Exclusive
6 months	Cereals	(soft cooked rice)
5-7 months	Vegetables and fruits (cooked and strained)	(potatoes, tomatoes, bananas)
6-8 months	Protein foods (cooked and strained)	meat, fish, chicken, beans, yogurt, egg
9-12 months	Start replacing strained fruits, vegetables and meat by addition of well-cooked, mashed or chopped vegetables, fruits and meat	meat, fish, chicken, beans, yogurt, egg

Guidelines For Feeding During The First Year Of Life (5,6)

Food Group	Major Nutrient Supplied	Amount	Serving Equivalence
Milk Milk, yogurt, cheese etc.	Protein Vitamin B2 & B12 Calcium	6 months: 30 oz of breast milk 6-9 months: 24 oz of breast milk 9-12 months: 16 -24 oz of breast milk	
Meat Mutton, beef, fish, chicken, beans etc.	Protein Vitamin B1& B5 Iron	6 months: none 6-8 months: 1-2 servings 9-12 months: 2 servings	1 serving= 1 oz meat, chicken, or fish; 1 egg; 1 cup cooked beans, peas, or lentils
Grain Breads, rice, porridge etc.	Carbohydrates VitaminB1 & B5 Iron	6 months: 1-2 servings 6-12 months: 2-3 servings 12 months: 4 servings	1 serving = • slice bread; • cup cooked rice or porridge
Fruits and Vegetables etc.	Carbohydrates Vitamins A & C	6 months: 1 serving fruit 6-8 months: 2 servings fruit,1-2 servings vegetable 9-12 months: 4 servings	1 serving = • piece of fruit, • cup cooked vegetables

GUIDELINES FOR FEEDING FROM FIRST– SIX YEARS OF LIFE (5,6)

Food Group	Major Nutrient Supplied	Amount/day	Age	Serving Equivalence
Milk Milk, yogurt, cheese etc.	Protein Vitamin B2 & B12 Calcium	4 servings	1-2 years	1 serving = • cup
			2-3 years	1 servings=' • - • cup
			3-4 years	1 servings= • - • cup
			4-5 years	1 servings=' • - • cup
			5-6 years	1 servings= • cup
Meat Mutton, beef, fish, poultry, beans etc.	Protein Vitamin B1 & B5 Iron	2-3 servings	1-2 years	1 serving= 2 Tbs of meat, chicken, fish; 1 egg; • cup of cooked beans, peas, or lentils
			2-3 years	1 serving= 3 Tbs of meat, chicken, fish; 1 egg; • cup of cooked beans, peas, or lentils
			3-4 years	1 serving= • cup of meat, chicken, fish; 1 egg; 1/3 cup of cooked beans, peas, or lentils
			4-5 years	1 serving= 1/3 cup of meat, chicken, fish; 1 egg; • cup of cooked beans, peas, or lentils
			5-6 years	1 serving= • cup of meat, chicken, fish; 1 egg; • • cup of cooked beans, peas, or lentils
Grain Breads, rice, porridge etc.	Carbohydrates VitaminB1 & B5 Iron	4 servings	1-2 years	1 serving = • slice bread; • cup cooked rice or porridge
			2-3 years	1 serving = 1 slice bread; • cup cooked rice or porridge
			3-4 years	1 serving = 1 slice bread; • cup cooked rice or porridge
			4-5 years	1 serving =1 slice bread; • cup cooked rice or porridge
			5-6 years	1 serving =1-2 slice bread; • cup cooked rice or porridge
Fruits and Vegetables etc.	Carbohydrates Vitamin A & C	4 servings to include 1 serving of vitamin A containing fruits/vegetables 1 serving of vitamin C containing fruits/vegetables 2 servings of other fruits	1-2 years	1 serving= • cup of fruit, • cup cooked vegetables
			2-3 years	1 serving= 1/3 cup of fruit, 1/3 cup cooked vegetables
			3-4 years	1 serving= • cup of fruit, • cup cooked vegetables
			4-5 years	1 serving= • cup of fruit, • cup cooked vegetables
			5-6 years	1 serving= 1 cup of fruit, 1 cup cooked vegetables

Birth to 36 months: Boys
Length-for-age and Weight-for-age percentiles

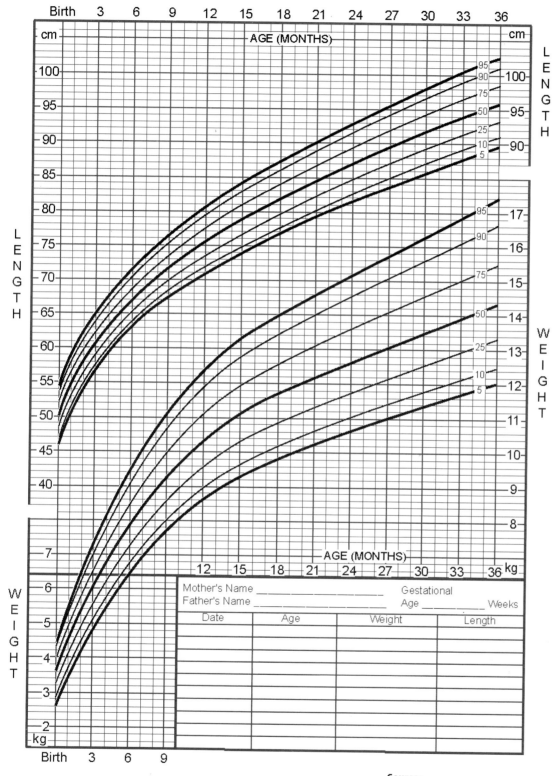

Source:
Source:
Modified and adapted with
permission from Centers for
Disease Control and
Prevention (CDC) USA, 2000.

Birth to 36 months: Girls
Length-for-age and Weight-for-age percentiles

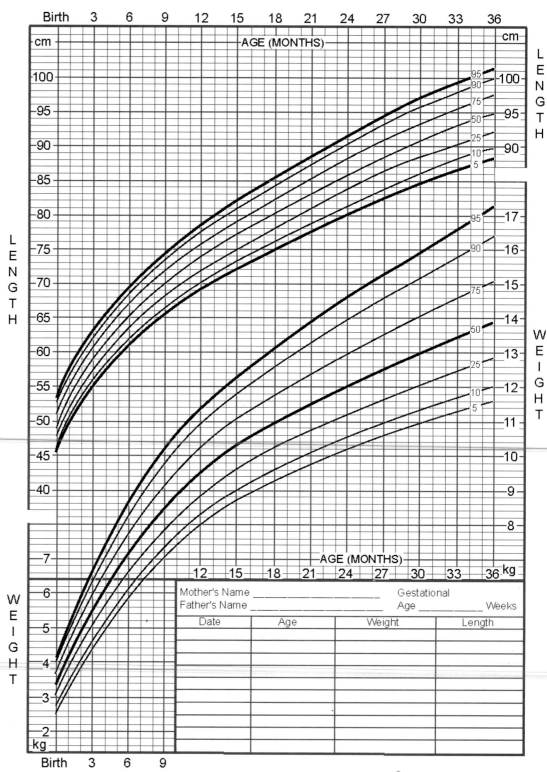

Source:
Modified and adapted with permission from Centers for Disease Control and Prevention (CDC) USA, 2000.

2 to 20 years: Boys
Stature-for-age and Weight-for-age percentiles

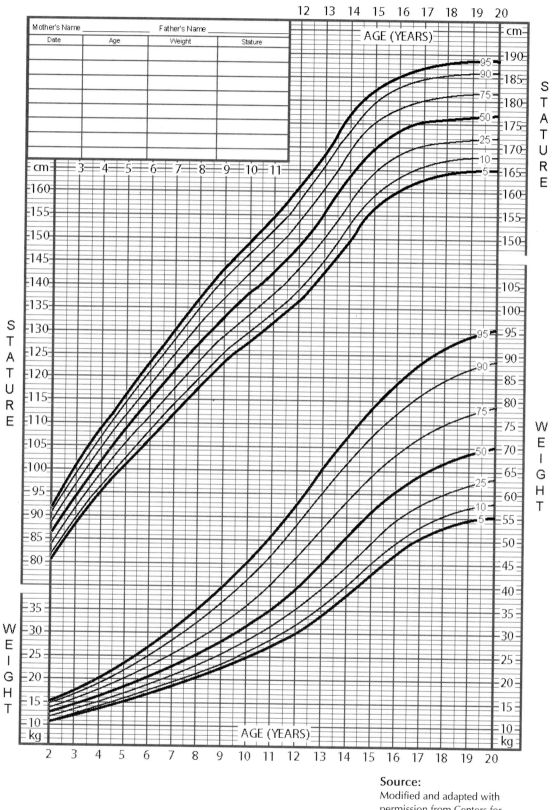

Source:
Modified and adapted with
permission from Centers for
Disease Control and
Prevention (CDC) USA, 2000.

2 to 20 years: Girls
Stature-for-age and Weight-for-age percentiles

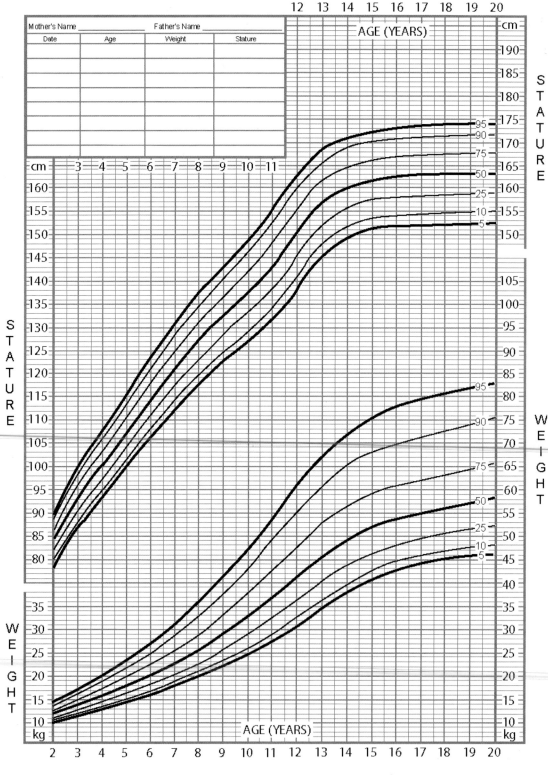

Source:
Modified and adapted with permission from Centers for Disease Control and Prevention (CDC) USA, 2000.

Specimen of a checklist for observation for home environment

CHECKLIST FOR OBSERVATION

STATISTICS CHECKLIST

Name of the child ....

Age　　　　　　 ....

Sex　　　　　　 Male　　　　 Female

Time　　　　　　 ....

Caregivers available　 Yes　　　　 No

Date of observation　 ....

Complete address ....

....

Observer's name...

Supervisor's name...

ACTION CHECKLIST (7)

Instruction:

Mark 'Yes' or 'No' in front of each observation

1	Parent tells the child, name of the (e.g., toys) object or person during visit	Yes	No
2	Parent spontaneously praises child at least twice	Yes	No
3	Parents do not shout at child during visit	Yes	No
4	Family has a pet	Yes	No
5	Parent provides toys to the child to play with, during the visit	Yes	No
6	Availability of muscle activity toys	Yes	No

Specimen of a Body of the Questionnaire

Child Development Research Questionnaire

Module I

Primary Caregiver is the respondent I will ask you some questions related to the birth of your youngest child

S. No.	Questions	Coding Categories	Skip to	Responses
1.1	What is the age of the child?	Specify Exact #		
1.2	How much was the period of pregnancy?	1. Full term 2. Premature 3. Post mature		
1.3	Where was this child delivered?	1. Home 2. Hospital		
1.4	By whom should a delivery be conducted?	1. Doctor 2. LHV 3. Midwife 4. Trained Dai 5. TBA 6. Others (Specify)		

Module II

Now, I will ask you some question related to the nutritional practice of your youngest child

S. No.	Questions	Coding Categories	Skip to	Responses
2.1	What should a newborn child be given as first feed?			
2.2	What was the first feed that this child was given?	1. Colostrum 2. Breastfeed 3. Honey 4. Cow's milk 5. Others (Specify)		
2.3	Did you breastfeed your youngest child?	1. Yes 2. No	If 2, Go to 2.5	
2.4	How long did you breastfeed?	Specify Exact #		

Name of Institution
Name of Department

Consent Form

Title of the project ....

Principal Investigator

Name: ....

Designation: ....

Department: ....

Introduction

GREETINGS

We belong to the __(Name of the institution)__ and are conducting a study about the social environment of children. We invite you to participate in this research study, the purpose of which is (for example) the study of factors in the social environment that affect learning ability in children aged less than three years. Before you can decide whether or not to volunteer to answer the questions for this study, you must understand the purpose of this study and how it may affect you. This consent form gives you information about the study, which will be discussed with you. Once you understand the purpose, and if you agree to participate, you will be asked to sign this informed consent form.

Purpose of the study

The purpose of this research is to identify the association between factors of social environment and physical growth, social behaviour and learning ability. Social environment broadly refers to factors that influence learning during early childhood with particular interest in sensory stimulation, economics and health.

Procedure

An interview using a questionnaire will be conducted, taking approximately 45-60 minutes of your time. Questions will be asked about your knowledge and practices as regards child rearing, and assessment of the child's developmental status will be done. No treatment or laboratory investigations are required. There is no risk involved to your physical and mental health. All information gathered in this study would be kept in the strictest confidence. Data collectors will be rigorously directed and monitored to keep the confidentiality of the study participants. All records will be identified by code numbers, and stored in a locked file cabinet. It will be the responsibility of the principal investigator to keep information about study participants confidential.

Your participation is voluntary and there will be no cost to you to participate in this study other than the time you spend with the interviewer. You will not receive any money or compensation or other reward for your participation. If you have any questions about the study, the Principal Investigator, __ (Name of Principal Investigator) __ will be glad to answer them.

Potential benefits

The findings of the study will help the government authorities, community health workers and community service providers to take steps to improve the current state of children at the community level, and will help them to design programs/strategies to enhance child development.

Your participation is voluntary. You are free to stop participating in the research at any time or decline to answer any specific questions without penalty.

Are you willing to give this interview?   Yes   No

I agree to participate in this study. I understand the information given to me, and I have received the answers to any questions I may have had about the research procedure. I understand and agree to the conditions of this study as described.

Respondent's name: ....

Signature / thumb impression of the respondent:...

Signature of the interviewer:...

INVESTIGATOR'S AFFIDAVIT

I certify that I have explained to the above individual(s) the nature and purpose of the study along with the potential benefits. I certify that the informed consent procedure has been followed, and that I have answered any questions from the participants above as fully as possible. I have answered any questions that have been raised and have witnessed the above signature on the date indicated below.

Name of the individual obtaining the consent: ....

Designation: ....

Signature   ....

Date   ....

Tel.# of the principal investigator in case of any inquiries/questions:

Child Development Research Questionnaire

Face Sheet

Respondent's Name: ....

Relation of the respondent with the child: ....

Name of Head of the Household: ....

Complete Address: ....

Date of Interview:

1st visit: ___/___/___   2nd visit: ___/___/___   3rd visit: ___/___/___

Interviewer's Name: ....

Supervisor's Name: ....

Checked by: ....

Edited by: ....

Steps to map out the study area

1.   Take a round of the whole of muhalla to be surveyed, and select a central point.
2.   Field staff will make sketches of all houses, starting from the central point of that locality.
3.   Draw all the buildings present in the area for example, mosques, school, well, streets and shops, corresponding to their place in the community.
4.   Completely transfer the landmarks of the whole area on paper.
5.   While making the sketch of the area, one member of the team should prepare a list of all the residents of each house, along with their age and gender. The house number in the list should correspond with the identification number on the map.

Framework of the Area

S. No.	Head of Household	No of < 3 years children	Address
1	Peer Bux	3	H#3,St#5,Baldia Town, Karachi
2	Salamat Ali	1	H#4,St#5 Baldia Town, Karachi
3	David Gill	2	H#3
4	Vikram Dharani	1	H#6

Early Childhood Development Program—Operational Plan and Time Line

Gantt Chart		Jan	Feb	Mar	Apr	May	Jun	Jul	Aug	Sep	Oct	Nov	Dec
	Activities	Dates												
1	Timelines													
2	Community Interaction													
	• Identification of repre-sentatives													
	• Formation of ECD committee													
3	Team selection													
4	Developing Training Material													
5	Training													
6	Development of project tools/material	.												
7	Project activities													
	• Center based activities													
	• Community based activities													
	• Health education for care givers													
	• Growth and development monitoring (follow up)													
	• Anthropometric assessment													
	• Observation of child													
	• Health indicators													
8	Project Material													
	• Requirements													
	• Purchase													
	• Availability													
9	Logistics													
10	Data management													
11	Report writing													
12	Information dissemination													
13	Feedback to the community													

Gantt chart can be modified in weeks or days according to requirements.

GLOSSARY

Chapter 1

Human Development: The process by which individuals families, social groups and populations generally progress towards achieving their potential level of physical, mental, social and economic health and well-being.

Prenatal: The process of growth and development from conception through birth, which spans approximately nine months. The prenatal period requires physical, medical and social care to achieve positive outcomes of pregnancy for the mother and her baby.

Infancy: Period includes the first two years of life. Infants are completely dependent on others, with limited prior knowledge and experience, but with eagerness to learn. Growth and development are most rapid during infancy.

Childhood, Early: Period includes first three to five years of life. Early childhood behaviour and development has a propensity to vary and move back and forth from time to time; language, reasoning and curiosity are rapidly acquired during toddler-hood. In the literature, especially regarding ECD Programming, the age groups in this period varies, and usually ranges from three to seven years. In this context, the book considers on average the first six years of life as period of early child development for all discussion purposes.

Childhood, Middle: Period includes from the sixth to eleventh year of life. Middle childhood has a remarkable capacity for memory, language, inquiry and social skills. For most children, it is also a phase of transition from home based to school based environment.

Adolescence, Early: Period includes from twelfth to fourteenth year of life. Early adolescence is the period of transition between childhood and adulthood.

Adolescence, Late: Period includes from fifteenth to nineteenth year of life. The formation of positive identity is an important psychosocial task. The late adolescents begin to make career choices, majority seek to complete their education, and enter the world of work.

Adulthood, Early: Period includes from twenty-first to thirty-ninth year of life. Achieving intimacy, making career choices, attaining vocational success are important challenges of early adulthood, and many decisions made during this period set the stage for later life.

Adulthood, Middle: Period includes from fortieth to fifty-ninth year of life.

Adulthood, Late: Period of life spans from sixtieth year onwards.

Development, Mental: The process of progression in the mental abilities of the child such as psychomotor, memory, language, thinking, reasoning, problem solving and curiosity.

Development, Emotional: The process of progression in the emotional abilities of the child such as attachment, trust, security, love, and affection, and a variety of emotions and feelings.

Development, Social: The process of progression in the social abilities of the child such as interactions with the individual and group through which he or she gets accustomed and influenced with the societal norms and values.

Socialization: The process by which persons develop understanding about general behaviour and customs of the society and groups; which help them to adjust and function within it or them.

Childcare: The pattern of behaviour and practices of caregivers; provision of food, health care, sensory stimulation and emotional support to the child.

Caregiver: Person who understands what children in general need, and fulfil their essential physical and psychological needs for healthy survival, growth and development. Usually caregivers are mother, father, sibling, relatives and childcare service providers (e.g. education and health personnel).

Primary caregiver: The main caregiver with a capacity to respond appropriately to the child's needs of feeding, sleeping, clothing, hygiene and one to one interactions.

Chapter 2

Social Environment: It comprises people, places, and things in the surroundings which mutually interact with the child.

Sensory Stimulation: Stimulus which influences any of the five senses of hearing, touch, smell, taste and sight. Social environment is the primary source of sensory stimulation to the child.

Sense, Auditory: Sense of hearing.

Sense, Tactile: Sense of touch.

Sense, Olfactory: Sense of smell.

Sense, Gustatory: Sense of taste.

Sense of Sight: Sense of vision.

Quality time (for the child): Period of the that caregivers give to the children in talking, playing, reading and disciplining, include ways of interaction that encourage children's expanding motor, cognitive and social skills.

Safe environment: Minimal or absolutely no indications of hazard of physical or psychosocial nature from the people, places, and things in the surroundings of the children.

Caregiver Involvement: Quality of being responsive assumes that caregiver understands the child's needs and responds promptly to it.

Learning Opportunities: Level of provision of age appropriate learning materials, as well as authorization to manipulate and play with them.

Chapter 3

Child assessment: It is the measurement of various aspects related to physical growth, behaviour and mental processes of the child, on the basis of specific standard criteria.

Screening: A preliminary assessment of the child for early identification of any developmental delay or growth faltering.

Test Materials: These comprise different objects that are required to conduct growth and development assessments.

Rapport: The term refers to familiarity and friendliness with a person or persons.

Personality: Overall distinctive, relatively stable patterns of each individual of reacting to and interacting with others.

Temperament: Emotional underpinning of personality, partially determined by genetics.

Activity Level: Predisposition of vigor and self-motivation as compared to passivity and immobility.

Irritability: Predisposition of moving angrily away from or towards new people, objects or experiences. It is an indication of negative emotionality.

Task Persistence: Predisposition of maintaining concentration and effort for an undertaking.

Child, Easy: Type of temperament; characterized by high levels of activity, approach and task persistence, and low levels of irritability, inhibition and anxiety.

Child, slow to warm: Type of temperament; characterized by high levels of persistence, approach, inhibition and anxiety task, and low levels of activity and irritability.

Child, Difficult: Type of temperament; characterized by high levels of activity and irritability, and low levels of task persistence, approach, inhibition and anxiety.

Chapter 4

Nutrition: Science of composition of nutrients of food and their effects on health.

Calorie: A unit of measure of the amount of energy supplied by food.

Nutrients: Chemical substances found in foods that are used by the body for growth and health.

Diet, Balanced: A diet that provides neither too much nor too little nutrients from all the categories.

Diet, Adequate: A diet consisting of foods that together supply sufficient protein, vitamins, and minerals and as many calories as necessary to meet a person's need.

Diet, Healthy: Diet characterized by balance, adequacy and variety of nutrients.

Malnutrition: Poor nutrition resulting from an excess or lack of calories or nutrients. Malnutrition early in life has long-term effects on mental and physical development.

Food security: Access at all times to an adequate supply of safe and nutritious foods.

Food insecurity: Inadequate or uncertain supply of safe and nutritious foods.

Physical growth: The process characterized by increase in body size.

Development: The process of progression in the functional capabilities of the body.

Failure to thrive: Any child who does not measure up to age appropriate growth and development standards.

Dietary supplements: Any commercial product of nutrients intended to supplement the day-to-day diet.

Iron deficiency: A disorder that results from a depletion of required iron reserves in the body.

Antenatal care: Care provided to a woman during pregnancy by trained and skilled health personnel such as doctors, nurses or midwives.

Colostrum: Yellowish milk produced during the first few days (usually first three days 3 or so) after delivery.

Weaning: Derived from word "wean", which means to discontinue breast-feeding and substitute other feeding habits. After six months, introduction of nutrient sources other than breast milk initiates weaning.

Food allergy: Unfavourable or adverse reaction to a normally harmless substance in food that involves the body's immune system. Variety of food causing allergy, changes with age and personal predisposition.

Anthropometry: The term anthropometry is made up of two words, i.e. 'Anthrop' means 'man' and 'metry' means 'measurement'. Hence, anthropometry is the measurement of the physical dimensions including size, weight, and proportions of different parts of the human body.

Anthropometric indices: These are a combination of body weight and height with consideration for age and sex of the child. Indices are expressed in terms of z-scores i.e. deviation of the observed value from the median value of the reference population, divided by the standard deviation of the reference population. Common indices are height for age, weight for height, and weight for age. They are categorized at the –2 SD cut-off levels to form the indicators stunting, under weight and wasting respectively.

Wasting (Weight-for-height): Anthropometrical Index; reflects body weight relative to height. If the child is gaining insufficient weight relative to height, or is losing weight, he or she comes under the label of low weight for height or wasting.

Stunting (Height-for-age): Anthropometrical Index; reflects whether the height is appropriate for age or not. If the child is gaining insufficient height relative to age it is referred to as stunting.

Underweight (Weight-for-age): Anthropometrical Index; reflects body mass relative to age. If the child is gaining insufficient weight relative to age, or is losing weight, that child is considered underweight.

Parameters of growth: Weight, height, head circumference and mid -upper arm circumference are the common growth parameters.

Length: Height measurement technique for infants is known as "Length"

Stature: Height measurement technique for children is known as "Stature",

Low birth weight: Infants born weighing less than 2500 grams (2.5 kg)

Growth Monitoring: The process of regular anthropometric measurement, recording and interpretation of a child's growth change.

Growth promotion: The regular process to use growth monitoring in order to counsel and enable the caregivers to increase control over and to improve the growth of their children.

Nutritional Counselling: The process by which one person helps another to clarify their concepts and understanding as well as guidance regarding food, diet and dietary practices.

Chapter 5

Intelligence: Person's ability to acquire, retain and understand different concepts, to understand the relationship between objects, events, and ideas, and as the ability to apply this understanding in solving the problems of everyday life.

Memory: It is the capacity of the mind to understand, store and retrieve information.

Language, Comprehension: The language that the child understands.

Language, Production: It consists of the words and combination of words the child uses.

Reasoning: A set of cognitive processes by which an individual may reach a conclusion based on presented instances.

Problem solving: A process of identifying and analyzing problems, discussing them and arriving at workable solutions, which can in turn be evaluated and improved in subsequent attempts.

Psychomotor: It is the skill that relates mental to muscular activity.

Psychomotor, Fine: Refers to small muscle movement and control; use of small muscle groups for specific tasks such as stacking small blocks, stringing beads, tracking an object with the eyes, smiling and handwriting.

Psychomotor, Gross: Refers to large muscle movement and control; use of large muscle groups for specific tasks such as holding your head up, walking, running, skipping, climbing, jumping.

Curiosity: Exploratory behaviour; the degree to which a child reacts to a new, strange and incongruous element in the environment. This could be by observing the object, approaching the object, manipulating the object and finally asking questions about the object.

Emotional state: This refers to the state of a person's emotions, especially with regard to pleasure or dejection.

Learning styles: Learning is a process of sensory perception and processing of information. Every individual has preferred sensory perceptions for it. Preferred perceptual modality for learning is considered as learning styles.

Learning, Auditory: Type of learning style; the child prefers auditory information, and retains content that has been verbally communicated.

Learning, Visual: Type of learning style; the child prefers visual depiction of the information; and learns through images, enjoys art and drawing, reads maps, charts and diagrams well.

Learning, Kinaesthetic- tactile: Type of learning style; the child prefers knowledge processes through physical sensations.

Learning Disability: A disorder which affects a child's ability to either adequately interpret what they see and hear, or to link the processed information from different parts of the brain.

Chapter 6

Observation: Observation is gathering information from the real world by recognizing and noting facts or behaviour as they occur.

Observation, Naturalistic: Type of observation based on setting; observation of behaviour in a natural setting, without any attempt by the observer to intervene.

Observation, Structured: Type of observation based on setting; purposeful intervening by the observer to cause an event to occur, or to set up a situation so that event can be more easily recorded.

Observation, Undisguised Participant: Type of observation based on observer; the individuals who are being observed know that the observer is present for the purpose of collecting information about their behaviour.

Observation, Disguised Participant: Type of observation based on observer; the individuals who are being observed do not know that the observer is present for the purpose of collecting information about their behaviour.

Checklist, Static: Type or portion of checklist; contains descriptions of the relatively permanent aspect of the subject or context being recorded.

Checklist, Action: Type or portion of checklist; contains descriptions of the presence or absence of specific behaviours being recorded.

Standardized approach: Criteria set to achieve consistency in the quality of the data collection especially with regard to setting, materials, language, prompting and total time spent.

Parent: An individual with short or long-term primary care giving responsibility for a child.

Parenting: Refers to the concept of managing the growth and development of the child.

Parenting Domains: Conventionally parenting has got four domains; control: clear provision of limit setting, discipline; nurturance: provision of food, cloth, shelter, warmth; maturity demands: expecting age appropriate behaviour; and communication: responsive aspect of parent – child interaction.

Parenting, Authoritative Style: Type of parenting style; characterized by high levels of control, nurturance, maturity demands and communication.

Parenting, Authoritarian style: Type of parenting style; characterized by high levels of control and maturity demands, while low levels of nurturance and communication.

Parenting, Permissive style: Type of parenting style; characterized by high levels of nurturance, while low levels of control, maturity demands and communication.

Parenting, Neglecting style: Type of parenting style; characterized by low levels of control, nurturance, maturity demands and communication.

Punishment: The practice of imposing something unpleasant on a wrongdoer.

Reinforcement: by rewarding the child.

Play: Act of occupying oneself in unrestrained, amusing interaction or recreation with people or things, which lead to voluntary or involuntary learning.

Play, Sensory Motor: Type of child's play; by approximately age 1, children spend most of their playtime in exploration and manipulation of objects provided to them

Play, Constructive: Type of child's play; by approximately age 2, children bring into play objects in the surroundings to construct things. Resourcefulness of the environment helps them to play more enthusiastically

Play, First Pretend: Type of child's play; by approximately age 2, children also initiate pretend or make believe play.

Play, Substitute Pretend: Type of child's play; by about age 2 to 3, children use items as a proxy for something different during play.

Play, Socio-dramatic: Type of child's play; by age 3 to 5 or so, children begin to act in role-plays

Chapter 7

Interview: A formal interaction between two or more people for the purpose of information gathering. Interviews vary in style and format.

Interview, Questionnaire based: Type of interview research based; the research interviewing technique which allows person-to-person formal conversation leading to information gathering based on predetermined structured questions and is formal in nature.

Interview, in depth: Type of research based interview; the research interviewing technique allows person to person discussion that leads to increased insight into people's thoughts, feelings and behaviours on respective issues. Questions are unstructured, based on guidelines and flexible in nature.

Questionnaire: A set of written questions used to collect data about opinions, attitudes, and knowledge from a person of interest.

Question, Closed-ended: Type of question; fixed number of response options, which allows the respondent to make a choice by choosing one of the listed options.

Question, Open Ended: Type of question; no predetermined set of responses, and the participant is free to answer.

Informed Consent: The consideration for each person's autonomy for the decision of complete, partial or no involvement, after understanding by him/her the nature and consequences of assessment or intervention process.

Sampling: Sampling is a process of selection of research participants among all eligible in the study population as per prescribed protocol.

Sampling unit: Eligible individual of the defined research population from whom information can be potentially collected.

Sampling Frame: List of all potential sampling units within the target population, from which sample will be actually drawn.

Sampling, Random: Type of sampling strategy; every eligible individual has an equal chance of being selected out of the study population.

Sampling, Systematic: Type of sampling strategy; selection of study participants from the study population according to some simple, systematic rule.

Pre-testing: The trial of the research instrument on a similar but not the same population on which final data will be collected.

Chapter 8

Focus Group Discussion: Carefully planned discussion designed to obtain perceptions of the participants in a defined area of interest, in a permissive and non-threatening environment moderated by a facilitator.

General Discussion: Casual dialogue among people on any topic without any moderation by a facilitator or without following any ground rules.

Group Interviewing: Emphasis is on interviewing a number of people simultaneously, based on questions from the researcher and specific responses from each member of the group.

Exploratory focus groups: Forum of focus group discussions regarding the caregiver's perception, understanding or even needs regarding child development.

Experiential focus groups: Forum of focus group discussions regarding caregiver's experiences, observation or even motivation level for potential and challenges regarding child development.

Deviance: Change from the normal or usual behavioural pattern.

Positive Deviance: Constructive deviation from the normal child rearing practices of the caregiver, resulting in more than expected growth and developmental status of the child.

Positive Deviant: Caregiver who is able to more effectively utilize existing resources in the environment, resulting in more than expected growth and developmental status of the child.

Maternal technology: Refers to practices, behaviours and beliefs of the caregiver related to handling of food and water, feeding pattern, personal hygiene, child care and interaction, sensory stimulation, safety and security.

Vulnerable: Children develop into psychologically ailing adults due to poor nurturing or traumatic early circumstances.

Resilient: Children develop into psychologically healthy adults despite poor nurturing or traumatic early circumstances.

Chapter 9

Communication: It refers to the sharing of thoughts, either in verbal or non-verbal ways.

Communication, Sender: A person who conveys a particular message.

Communication, Receiver: A person who receives the message and comprehends its meaning.

Communication, Message: The content of the communication, which is to be sent from one person to another person.

Communication, Verbal: System of communication; uses spoken words to convey the message.

Communication, Nonverbal: System of communication; includes facial expression, body movements, and gestures to convey the message. Also commonly referred as body language.

Communication, Language of:
Composition of words people use to share ideas and experiences with others.

Communication, Paralinguistic Features: Features of a spoken message that is not contained in the words alone i.e. rhythm, pace, emphasis, intonation, pitch and tone of voice.

Communication, Body Language: Communication via the movements or attitudes of the body.

Communication, Posture: A characteristic way of positioning the body or its parts; implicitly conveys a person's emotional or mental state.

Counselling: The process employed by the professional or paraprofessional worker (counsellor) to help caregivers clarify their issues related to child care and to decide upon further lines of action.

Counselling, Prescriptive: Type of counselling; refers to the counsellor's intention of recommending a particular solution or line of action related to child care.

Counselling, Informative: Type of counselling; refers to the counsellor's intention to give additional information or education to the caregiver for situations related to child care.

Counselling, Process: Conventionally, counselling has three stages; problem identification: clarification of issues related to child care practices, goal-setting: selection of preferred child care practices, and action: moving towards the preferred child care practices.

Chapter 10

Community: Refers to a group which has some common characteristics. This generally means a common culture, language, common interests and identity, common set of values and beliefs.

Community Dynamics: From the ECD perspective, it is a specific pattern of child rearing practices and traditions, and value different knowledge and skills expected from the child at community level.

Social Class: Relative economic and social positions within any given society. For individual families, the designation is based on the income, occupation, area of residence and education of the adults in the household

Community, Farm-Based: Type of inhabited community; livelihood is generally linked to harvesting and cultivating available natural resources through farming, fishing, raising livestock, etc.

Community, non-Farm-Based: Type of inhabited community; livelihood is generally linked to the manufacturing and service oriented sectors, and families have greater access to manufactured products.

Community Orientation: From ECD perspective, learning about a particular community in terms of geographical boundaries, demographics, cultural and religious value system, mother and child status, sources of income, key people and leaders, concerns in relation to child development, assurance and readiness for involvement in ECD programme activities, potential partners and competitors for ECD endeavours.

Chapter 11

ECD Programme: Network of individuals assist in identification of Early Childhood Care needs in a community, and allows the community to take an active role in developing and advocating programs suited to those needs. Research components of such programs are systematic and purposeful investigations for early childhood problems, to identify reasons relating to these problems.

Community Based: Comprehensive provision of care in homes and communities to children from birth to six years of age, based on an integrated approach to augment nutrition, health and therapeutic services, promotion of developmental opportunities, and provision of other social services.

ECD Programme, Planning cycle: A methodical plan that identifies ECD needs, selects the best way to meet the identified needs, implements the methods and evaluates the extent to which those needs are met for future plan of action.

ECD Programme, Community Developmental: Create and support network of individuals to assist programmes in early childhood care in a community. This allows the community to take an active role in developing and advocating activities suited to their own needs and providing a favourable environment for ECD. These programmes can have components of research as well.

ECD Programme, Research: Systematic and purposeful investigations for early childhood problems to identify reasons relating to these problems. Conventionally, the service provision element is not included in ECD research programmes.

ECD Programme, Sustainability: Capability of an ECD programme ensuring continuity of its initiatives for an extended period of time through efficient use of resources, commitment and provision of services by involving the community.

ECD Programme, Situation Analysis: Evaluation of the present situation from the perspective of parents, education and health care service providers, and the community as a whole. It is also possible to collect information regarding awareness and motivation level of community members in the context of ECD.

ECD Programme, Needs Assessment: Systematic appraisal of a community to evaluate its ECD related requirements. The purpose is to set priorities for future actions or programme design.

ECD Related Social Services: Miscellaneous services are required at community level to provide a conducive environment for child development. From the health care sector it includes dispensaries, hospitals, doctors, paramedical staff and medicines. From the education sector it includes schools and trained teachers. From the public works sector it includes safe water, sewage system, electricity and natural gas, and play area. From the social welfare sector it includes an ambulance service and shelter for the homeless, etc.

ECD Programme, Priority Setting: Prioritize child's needs for optimal growth and development for the respective community. This also gives the opportunity of prioritizing the programme according to existing facilities in the community in terms of materials, human and other resources.

ECD Programme, Strategy: Choosing a method and carrying it out to meet the set ECD objectives.

ECD Programme, Planning: Developing a work plan for implementation of strategies to achieve ECD objectives within a given timeframe.

Life cycle approach: ECD does not start from the child, rather it begins from the mother whom physical and mental health even prior to conception has a direct influence on later foetal development and child birth. Low birth weight babies are more likely to have a childhood of impaired development and poor physical health, giving rise to stunted adolescents with compromised physical and mental capabilities. Consequently as adults, they have reduced capacity to produce healthy babies and provide care to them. This creates a vicious circle that needs to be broken. A sound situation analysis will give relevant information on what stage an intervention is required in a particular community.

ECD Programme Design: It is an organized framework of specific information, giving details of selected community based strategies and a timeframe for ECD programme implementation.

Chapter 12

ECD Projects: Planned course of action with specific work plans to achieve ECD objectives.

Community, Participation: Contribution of members of the community to participate in joint situation analysis and ECD programme planning, which leads to action plans that can be transformed into a sustainable positive change in the ECD status of a community.

Community, Mobilization:
A process through which people in a community can be given common goals with the purpose of enabling them to work together, without prejudice or like and dislike for other members of the group.

Leadership: Capacity to influence the ideology and actions of the community, through the process of persuasion, towards achievement of a common goal.

ECD Field Coordinator: A community based ECD programme management position; responsible for coordination of the ongoing development and implementation process of an ECD Programme.

ECD Programme Manager: An ECD programme management position; responsible for planning, organizing, and directing resources for the community, through the process of administration and supervision, towards achievement of common ECD goals.

ECD Programme, Monitoring: Systematic process of checking and documenting ECD programme performance on an ongoing basis, involving programme process and outcomes.

ECD Programme, Evaluation: Systematic process to assess the extent to which ECD programmes meet objectives.

REFERENCES

Chapter 1
Fundamentals of Child Development

1.   Rice PF. *Human development: A life span approach.* 3rd ed. New Jersey: Prentice Hall; 1998; p. 7-9.

2.   Papalia ED, Olds Ws. *Human development.* 3 rd ed. New York: McGraw- Hill; 1986; p. 8-9.

3.   Santrock WJ. *Life- span development.* 8th ed. New York: McGraw-Hill Education; 2002; p.16-18.

4.   Thelen E. Learning to walk: Ecological demands and phylogenetic constraints. In Lipsitt LP, Rovee-Collier C., editors. *Advances in infancy research.* (Vol.3). Norwood, NJ: Ablex; 1984.

5.   Cole M, Cole RS. *The development of children.* 2nd ed. New York: Scientific American Books; 1993; p. 179.

6.   Thelen E, Ulrich BD, Jensen JL. The developmental origins of locomotion. In Woollacott M, Shumway-Cook A, editors. *The development of posture and gait across the lifespan.* Columbia: University of South Carolina Press; 1989.

7.   Tanner JM. Fetus into man: *Physical growth from conception to maturity.* Cambridge: Harvard University Press; 1978.

8.   Hetherinton ME, Parke DR. *Child psychology: A contemporary viewpoint.* 5 th ed. Boston: McGraw-Hill College; 1999; p. 180.

9.   Berk EL. *Infants, children and adolescents.* 2nd ed. Boston: Allyn and Bacon; 1996; p. 170.

10. Cole M, Cole RS. *The development of children.* 2nd ed. New York: Scientific American Books; 1993; p. 202.

11. Bowlby J. *Attachment and loss: Vol 1. Attachment.* London: Hogarth; 1969

12. Kochanska G. Patterns of inhibition to the unfamiliar in children of normal and affectively ill mothers. *Child Development* 1991; 61: 1934-1943.

13. Main M, Cassidy J. Categories of responses in union with the parents at age six: Predictable from infant attachment classifications and stable over a 1-month period. *Developmental Psychology* 1998; 24: 415-426.

14. Cole M, Cole RS. *The development of children.* 2nd ed. New York: Scientific American Books; 1993; p. 356.

15. Lucas A, Morley RC, Cole TJ. Randomised trial of early diet in preterm babies and later intelligence quotient. *British Medical Journal* 1998; 317: 1481-1487.

16.   Ahmed NU, et al. A longitudinal study of the impact of behaviour change intervention on cleanliness, diarrhoeal morbidity and growth of children in rural Bangladesh. *Social Science and Medicine* 1993; 37: 159-171.

17.   Baumrind D. Child care practices anteceding three patterns of preschool behaviour. **Genetic Psychology Monograph** 1967; 75: 43-88.

18.   LeMonda - Tamis CS, Bornstein MH. Habituation and maternal encouragement of attention in infancy as predictors of toddler language, play, and representational competence. *Child Development* 1989; 60: 738-751.

19.   Teller DY. First glances. The vision of infants. The Friedenwald Lecture. *Investigative Ophthamology & Visual Science* 1997; 38: 2183-2203.

Chapter 2
Social Environment

1.   Cole M, Cole RS. *The development of children*. 2nd ed. New York: Scientific American Books; 1993; p. 129.

2.   Berk EL. *Infants, children and adolescents*. 2nd ed. Boston: Allyn and Bacon; 1996; p. 158.

3.   Cole M, Cole RS. *The development of children*. 2nd ed. New York: Scientific American Books; 1993; p. 24.

4.   Hetherinton ME, Parke DR. *Child psychology: A contemporary viewpoint*. 5 th ed. Boston: McGraw-Hill College; 1999; p. 25-27.

5.   Bronfenbrenner U. *The ecology of human development*. Cambridge: Harvard University Press; 1979.

6.   Berk EL. *Infants, children and adolescents*. 4th ed. Boston: Allyn and Bacon; 2002; p. 29.

Chapter 3
General Guidelines for Child Assessment

1.   Anastasi A. *Psychological testing*. 5th ed. New York: Macmillan Publishing Co.; 1982; p. 22-44.

2.   Groth -Marnet G. *Handbook of psychological assessment*. 2nd ed. New York: John Wiley & Sons; 1990; p. 40-41.

3.   Bayley N. *Bayley scale of infant development*. 2nd ed.. California: Institute of human development; 1969.

4.   Frieberg LK. *Human development: Life span approach*. 4th ed. Boston: Jones and Bartlett Publishers;

1992. p.136-138.

5.   Bee H. *The developing child.* 9th ed. Boston: Allyn and Bacon; 2000; 97-99.

6.   Santrock WJ. *Life- span development.* 8th ed. New York: McGraw Hill Education; 2002; p. 182-184.

Chapter 4
Nutrition, Growth and Anthropometry

1.   Bender DA, Bender AE. *Bender's dictionary of nutrition and food technology.* 7th ed. Cambridge: Woodhead Publishing Limited; 1999.

2.   Ensminger A, Esminger ME, Konlande JE, Robson JR.. T*he concise encyclopedia of food and nutrition.* Florida: CRC Press; 1995.

3.   Tull A. *Food and Nutrition.* 3rd ed. Oxford: Oxford University Press; 1996.

4.   Wardlaw GM, Insel PM. *Perspectives in nutrition.* 2nd ed. St. Louis: Mosby; 1993.

5.   Williams SR. *Essentials of nutrition and diet therapy.* 6th ed. St. Louis: Mosby; 1994.

6.   United Nations' Children Fund. *The state of the world's children 2003.* NY: United Nations' Children Fund; 2003.

7.   Rivera JA, Martorell R, Ruel MT, Habichat JP, Hass JD. Nutritional Supplementation during the pre school years influences body size and composition of Guatemalan Adolescents. Journal of Nutrition. 1995; 125: 1068 S -77S.

8.   Brown JE. *Nutrition now.* 3rd ed. Belmont, CA: Wadsworth; 2002.

9.   World Health Organization. *Guidelines for training community health workers in nutrition.* Geneva: World Health Organization; 1981.

10.   Robinson CH, Lawler MR. *Normal and therapeutic nutrition.* 16th ed. NY: Macmillan Publishing Co; 1982.

11.   Behrman RE, Kliegman RM, Arvin AN. *Nelson textbook of pediatrics.* 15th ed. Philadelphia: W.B. Saunders Company; 1996.

12.   Pakistan Pediatric Association. *Textbook of pediatrics.* Lahore: Pakistan Pediatric Association; 2000.

13.   Carlson NR. *Foundations of physiological psychology.* 4th ed. MA: Allyn & Bacon; 1999.

14.   World Health Organization. *Physical Status: the use and interpretation of anthropometry. Report of a WHO expert committee.* Geneva: World Health Organization; 1995.

15.   United Nations Children's Fund. *Monitoring progress towards the goals of the world summit for children: A practical handbook for multiple –indicator surveys.* Planning Office, Evaluation and

Research Office Programme Division. New York: United Nations Children's Fund; 1995.

16.   http://www.hrsa.gov (accessed on March 18, 2004.).

17.   Illyas M. *Textbook of community medicine & public health*. 5th ed. Karachi: Time Publishers; 2000.

18.   http://www.cdc.gov (accessed on January 12, 2004).

19.   Young ME, editor. *Early child development: Investing in our children's future*. Proceedings of a World Bank Conference on Early Child Development: Investing in the future, Atlanta, Georgia; 1996 Apr 8-9; Washington, DC, USA. Amsterdam: Elsevier; 1997.

Chapter 5
Intellectual Assessment

1.   Myers GD. *Exploring psychology*. 3rd ed. New York: Worth Publishers; 1996; p. 275

2.   Rice PF. *Human development: A life span approach*. 3rd ed. New Jersey: Prentice Hall; 1998; p. 182-183.

3.   Myers GD. *Exploring psychology*. 3rd ed. New York: Worth Publishers; 1996; p. 264-268.

4.   Atkinson LR, Atkinson CR, et al. *Hilgard's introduction to psychology*. 12th ed. Orlando: Harcourt Brace & Company; 1996; p. 303-304.

5.   Gardner H. *Multiple intelligences: The theory in practice*. New York: Basic Books; 1993; p.281.

6.   Berry JW, Bennett JA. Conceptions of cognitive competence. *International Journal of Psychology* 1992; 27: 77-88.

7.   Myers GD. *Exploring psychology*. 3rd ed. New York: Worth Publishers; 1996; p. 285-288.

8.   Rice PF. *Human development: A life span approach*. 3rd ed. New Jersey: Prentice Hall; 1998; p. 197-198.

Chapter 6
Observational methodology

1.   Frieberg LK. *Human development: Life span approach*. 4th ed. Boston: Jones and Bartlett Publishers; 1992. p.16.

2.   Cole M, Cole RS. *The development of children*. 2nd ed. New York: Scientific American Books; 1993; p. 24.

3.   Shaughnessy JJ, Zechmeister BE. *Research methods in psychology*. 3 rd ed. New York: McGraw-Hill; 1994; p.75-95.

4.   Frieberg LK. *Human development: Life span approach*. 4th ed. Boston: Jones and Bartlett Publishers;

1992. p. 18.

5.   Clarke -Stewart, Alison PM, Friedman S. *Life long development*. New York: John Wiley & Sons; 1988; p. 36-39.

6.   Streubert JH, Carpenter RD. *Qualitative research in nursing: Advancing the humanistic imperative*. Philadelphia: J. B. Lippincott Company; 1995; 98-99.

7.   Patton QM. *Qualitative evaluation and research methods*. 2nd ed. Newbury Park, CA: SAGE Publications; 1990; 25-27.

8.   Babbie E. *The practice of social research*. 9th ed. Belmont, CA: Wadsworth/Thomson Learning; 2001; 295-298.

9.   Sharman C, Cross W, Vennis D. Observing children: A practical guide. 2nd ed. London: Cassell; 2000.

10. Berk EL. *Infants, children and adolescents*. 4 th ed. Boston: Allyn and Bacon; 2002; p. 396-398.

11. Frieberg LK. *Human development: Life span approach*. 4th ed. Boston: Jones and Bartlett Publishers; 1992. p.138

12. Santrock WJ. *Life- span development*. 8th ed. New York: McGraw Hill Education; 2002; p. 260-264

Chapter 7
Questionnaire-based interviews

1.   Zanden WVJ. *Human development*. 3rd ed. New York: Alfred A. Knopf; 1985; p. 39-40.

2.   Kvale S. Interviews: *An introduction to qualitative research interviewing*. Thousand Oaks, California: SAGE Publications; 1996

3.   Polit FD, Hungler PB. *Essentials of nursing research: Method, appraisal and utilization*. 3rd ed. Philadelphia: J.B. Lippincott Company; 1993; p. 200-206.

4.   Dempsey AP, Dempsey DA. *Nursing research with basic statistical applications*. 3rd ed. Boston: Jones and Bartlett Publishers; 1992; p. 39-43.

5.   Craig RJ, Metze PL. *Methods of psychological research*. 2 nd ed. Monterey, California: Brooks/ Cole Publishing Company; 1986; p. 167-171.

6.   Dempsey AP, Dempsey DA. *The research process in nursing*. California: Wadsworth Health Sciences; 1981; p. 74-82.

7.   Knapp RT. *Quantitative nursing research*. Thousand Oaks, California; 1998; p. 103-112.

8.   Crookes AP, Davis S, editors. Research into practice: Essential skills for reading and applying research

in nursing and health care. London: Bailliere Tindall; 1998; p. 143.

9. Sapsford R, abbott P. *Research methods for nurses and the caring professions*. Buckingham: Open University Press; 1994; p. 111- 112.

10. Polit FD, Hungler PB. *Essentials of nursing research: Method, appraisal and utilization*. 3rd ed. Philadelphia: J.B. Lippincott Company; 1993; p. 244-245.

Chapter 8
Focus Group Discussions

1. Morgan D. *Focus groups as qualitative research*. Newbury Parks, CA: SAGE Publication; 1988.

2. Kreuger RA. *Focus groups: A practical guide for applied research*. London: SAGE Publication; p. 18

3. Morse MJ. Editor. *Critical issues in qualitative research methods*. Thousand Oaks, California: SAGE Publications; 1994; p. 226-240

4. Patton QM. *How to use qualitative methods in evaluation*. Newbury Park, CA: SAGE Publications; 1987; p. 135-142.

5. Vaughn S, Schumm SJ, Sinagub J. *Focus group interviews in education and psychology*. Thousand Oaks: SAGE Publications; 1996.

6. Krueger R. *Focus groups: A practical guide for applied research*. Newbury Park, CA: SAGE Publications; 1987; p. 135-142.

7. Zeitlin M, Ghassemi H, Mansoor M. *Positive deviance in child nutrition with emphasis on psychosocial and behavioral aspects and implications for development* [online]. 1990 [cited 2004 Sep. 9] Available from: URL: http://www.unu.edu/unupress/unupbooks/80697e/80697E01.htm

Chapter 9
Communication Skills

1. Arnold E, Boggs K. *Interpersonal relationship: Professional communication skills for nurses*. Philadelphia: W. B. Saunders Company; 1989; p.13.

2. Devito AJ. *Essentials of human communication*. 2nd ed. New York: HarperCollins Publishers; 1996; p. 7-21.

3. Ellis BR, Gates JR, Kenworthy N, editors. *Interpersonal communication in nursing: Theory and practice*. Edinburgh: Churchill Livingstone; 1995; p. 4-8.

4. Ellis BR, Gates JR, Kenworthy N, editors. *Interpersonal communication in nursing: Theory and practice*. Edinburgh: Churchill Livingstone; 1995; p. 7-14.

5. Gorden LR. *Interviewing: Strategy, techniques and tactics.* 3rd ed. Illinios: The Dorsey Press; 1980; p. 213-232.

6. Nelson -Jones R. *Introduction to counseling skills: Text and activities.* London: SAGE Publication Ltd; 2000; p. 213-225.

7. Sundeen JS, Stuart WG, Rankin DAE, Cohen AS. *Nurse-client interaction: Implementing the nursing process.* 5th ed. St.Louis: Mosby- Year Book; 1994; p. 116-131.

Chapter 10
Community Dynamics

1. Mayers R. *The twelve who survive strengthening program of early child.* 2nd ed. Michigan: High/Scope Press; 1995.

2. Taga A H. *Sociology: An introduction.* Lahore: 2000

3. Wadud E. Eds. Schultz J, Berkowitz B. *Community tool box: Recognizing allies.* Part I, Chapter 30, Section 4. Available from URL: http://ctb.ku.edu/tools/en/chapter_1030.htm . Last accessed: Nov 03, 2006

4. Vilela M, Nagy J, Fawcett SB. Ed Axner M. *Community tool box: Identifying targets and agents of change; who can benefit, who can help.* Part F, Chapter18, Section 3. Available from URL: http://ctb.ku.edu/tools/en/sub_section_main_1145.htm . Last accessed: Nov 03, 2006

5. Hampton C, Heaven C. Eds. Schultz J, Axner M. *Community toolbox: Understanding and describing the community.* Part B, Chapter 3, Section 2. Available from URL: http://ctb.ku.edu/tools/en/sub_section_main_1020.htm . Last accessed: Nov 03, 2006

Chapter 11
ECD Program Development

1. Shore R. *Rethinking the brain: New insights into early development.* New York, NY: Families and Work Institute. (Revised 10/03) 1997.

2. Rogers B L. *Health and economic consequences of malnutrition.* Available from URL: www.tulane.edu/~internut/publications/WB_Bckgrd_Pprs/Narrative/NarrativetwoRogers.doc

3. Anderson L M., Shinn C, Fullilove M T, Scrimshaw S C, Fielding J E, Normand J, Carande-Kulis V G and the Task Force on Community Preventive Services. Recommendations to promote healthy social environments. *American Journal of Preventive Medicine* 2003;24(3S)

4. Anderson L M., Shinn C, Fullilove M T, Scrimshaw S C, Fielding J E, Normand J, Carande-Kulis V G and the Task Force on Community Preventive Services. The effectiveness of early childhood development programs: A systematic review. *American Journal of Preventive Medicine* 2003;24(3S)

5. Tenenbaum I M. *A longitudinal research report on the early childhood development program.* South Carolina Department of Education. December 2000.

6. Park K. *Health planning and management: Park's textbook of preventive and social medicine.* 21st ed. Banarsidas Bhanot Publishers, India, 2001; 593-610

7. *A guide to social analysis for projects in developing countries.* Social development department: Overseas Development Administration, London, HMSO, 1995.

8. Heaver R A, Hunt J M. *Improving early childhood development: An integrated program for the Philippines.* The International Bank for Reconstruction and Development, the World Bank and the Asian Development Bank. November 1995

9. Thompson J, Kahn T, Masheder M, Oldfield L, Glockler M, Meighan R. *Fitting into society: Natural childhood.* Simon and Schuster Inc, New York, 1994, p. 100-111

10. Bronfenbrenner U. *The ecology of human development.* Harvard University Press: Cambridge, Massachusetts: 1979, p. 22-27.

11. *Early childhood development: Program designs, The World Bank Group.* Available form URL: http://www.worldbank.org/children/programdesign/progdes2.html . Last accessed Nov 03, 2006.

12. Evans J L, Myers R G, Ilfeld E M. *Early childhood counts: A programming guide on early childhood care for development.* The International Bank for Reconstruction and Development/World Bank, Washington DC, May 2000.

13. Simon J, Rosen S, Claeson M, Breman A, Tulloch J. *The family health cycle: From concept to implementation.* The International Bank for Reconstruction and Development / The World Bank 1818 H Street, NW, Washington, DC 20433. October 2001.

14. Kamal S. *A handbook on project development.* Pathfinder International. Karachi 1991

15. Yusof K, Batumalai S, Lin W Y, Okamura J. *The ABCs of community participation in primary health care.* Department of Publications, University of Malaya, Kuala Lumpur, 1989.

Chapter 12
ECD Projects Management

1. Evans J L, Myers R G, Ilfeld E M. *Early childhood counts: A programming guide on early childhood care for development.* The International Bank for Reconstruction and Development/World Bank, Washington DC, May 2000.

2. McMahon R, Barton E, Piot M. *What is management: On being in charge; a guide to management in primary health care.* 2nd Ed.WHO Geneva; p11-28,

3. Oakley P. *Projects with people: The practice of participation in rural development.* Oxford & IBH Publishing, New Delhi, 1993.

4.   Yusof K, Batumalai S, Lin W Y, Okamura J. T*he ABCs of community participation in primary health care.* Department of Publications, University of Malaya, Kuala Lumpur, 1989.

5.   Bhatnagar B, Williams A C. *Participatory development and the World Bank: Potential directions for change.* The International Bank for Reconstruction and Development/The World Bank Washington DC: World Bank Discussion Paper No 183. 1992

6.   Mayo M, Craig G. *Community participation: A reader in participation and development.* Zed Books Ltd London, 1995.

7.   Axner M. Berkowitz B. *Community toolbox: Core functions in leadership; learning how to be a community leader.* Part E, Chapter14, Section 1.Available from URL: http://ctb.ku.edu/tools/en/chapter_1014.htm . Last accessed: Nov 03, 2006.

8.   *Asmara declaration on early child development: Framework for action.* 2nd International Conference on Early Child Development October 28-31, 2002. Available from URL: www.adeanet.org/publications/docs/ASMARA%20Conference%20Overview%20Synt . Last accessed: Nov 03, 2006

9.   Rossi P H, Freeman H E, Lipsey M W. *Evaluation: A systematic approach.* 6th ed. Sage Publications: California; 1999.

10.   Perelman L C, Paradis J, Barrett E. *Document types: The Mayfield handbook of technical and scientific writing.* California: Mayfield publishing company: 1998, p. 39-174

11.   Bankowski Z, Ed. *General ethical principles: International guidelines for ethical review of epidemiological studies.* Council for International Organizations of Medical Sciences, Geneva, 1991. ISBN 92 9036 048 8. Sw.fr. 6 Available from URL: http://www.cioms.ch/frame_menu_texts_of_guidelines.htm . Last accessed: Nov 03, 2006.

Appendices:

1.   Bayley N*., Bayley Scale of Infant Development.* 2nd ed. California: Institute of Human Development;1969.

2.   Hetherinton M.E., Parke DR. Child psychology: *A contemporary viewpoint.* 5 th ed. Boston: McGraw Hill College; 1999.

3.   Berk E.L., *Infants, children and adolescents.* 2nd ed. Boston: Allyn and Bacon; 1996.

4.   Wardlaw G.M., Insel P.M., *Perspectives in nutrition.* 2nd ed. St. Louis: Mosby; 1993.

5.   Williams S.R., *Essentials of nutrition and diet therapy.* 6th ed. St. Louis: Mosby; 1994.

6.   Behrman R.E., Kliegman R.M., Arvin A.N., *Nelson textbook of pediatrics.* 15th ed. Philadelphia: W.B.Saunders Company; 1996.

7.   Adapted from: Caldwell B.M., Bradley R.H., *Administration manual: Home Observation for Measurement of the Environment.* Lit Rock, AR: University of Arkansas at Little Rock; 2003.

INDEX